More praise for Zoe Weil's

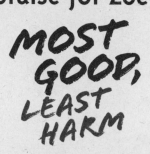

MOST GOOD, LEAST HARM

"Whether you're an educator, parent, or concerned citizen seeking practical tools for a more aligned, purposeful, and fulfilling life, *Most Good, Least Harm* offers clear and accessible pathways and insights for getting there.

Zoe Weil offers potent medicine for the false and commonly held belief that doing good requires personal sacrifice, and points the way to a path filled with congruence, reminding us that our inner and outer worlds are inextricably intertwined."

—Nina Simons, copresident and cofounder, Bioneers

"In a society where we often see ourselves as powerless to effect change, Zoe Weil provides a brilliant framework for leading us to a life of mindful choices, compassionate action, and collective change. *Most Good, Least Harm* is a guide to blending spiritual activism, moral self-reflection, and environmental concern for a more conscious life and a healthier planet."

—Gregg Krech, author of *Naikan: Gratitude, Grace, and the Japanese Art of Self-Reflection*

"Zoe Weil's pioneering book, *Most Good, Least Harm,* offers a vision for how we cultivate a loving sense of appreciation for all forms of life. With a rare blend of wit, wisdom, and humility, she offers an inspiring roadmap for how to lead our lives in a way which brings balance to ourselves and the planet."

—Susan Feathers, executive director, John and Terry Levin Center for Public Service and Public Interest Law— Stanford Law School

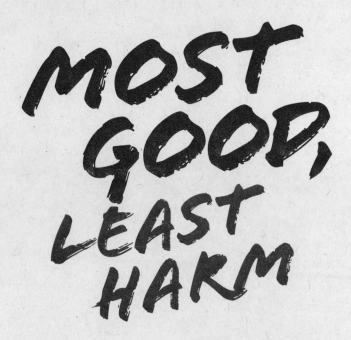

MOST GOOD, LEAST HARM

**A Simple Principle for a Better
World and Meaningful Life**

ZOE WEIL

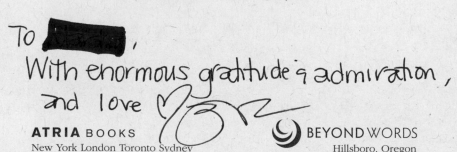

To ▮▮▮,
With enormous gratitude & admiration,
and love

ATRIA BOOKS
New York London Toronto Sydney

BEYOND WORDS
Hillsboro, Oregon

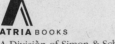

ATRIA BOOKS
A Division of Simon & Schuster, Inc.
1230 Avenue of the Americas
New York, NY 10020

BEYOND WORDS
20827 N.W. Cornell Road, Suite 500
Hillsboro, Oregon 97124-9808
503-531-8700 / 503-531-8773 fax
www.beyondword.com

Managing editor: Lindsay S. Brown
Editor: Julie Knowles
Copyeditor: Meadowlark Publishing Services
Proofreader: Jennifer Weaver-Neist
Design: Sara Blum
Composition: William H. Brunson Typography Services

First Atria Books/Beyond Words trade paperback edition January 2009

ATRIA BOOKS and colophon are trademarks of Simon & Schuster, Inc.
Beyond Words Publishing is a division of Simon & Schuster, Inc.

For more information about special discounts for bulk purchases,
please contact Simon & Schuster Special Sales at 1-800-456-6798 or
business@simonandschuster.com.

Manufactured in the United States of America

10 9 8 7 6 5 4 3 2 1

Library of Congress Cataloging-in-Publication Data:

Weil, Zoe.
    Most good, least harm : a simple principle for a better world and a meaningful life /
Zoe Weil.
        p. cm.
1. Conduct of life. 2. Change (Psychology). I. Title.
BJ1581.2.W368 2009
170'.44—dc22

2008037163

ISBN-13: 978-1-58270-206-3
ISBN-10:   1-58270-206-3

The corporate mission of Beyond Words Publishing, Inc.: *Inspire to Integrity*

For the generations of all people and all species to follow,
but especially for Forest.

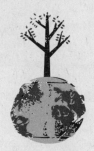

Contents

Contents

PART III
GETTING STARTED

... The salvation of the human world lies nowhere else than in the human heart, in the human power to reflect, in human modesty, and in human responsibility.
Vaclav Havel

As soon as you notice the slightest sign of indifference, the moment you become aware of the loss of a certain seriousness, of longing, of enthusiasm and zest, take it as a warning. Your soul suffers if you live superficially.
Albert Schweitzer

It just seems our species is happier when we are good.

Goodness is not guaranteed. A life of principle requires practice. ...
from *Unless*, a novel by Carol Shields

If there is any kindness I can show, or any good thing I can do to any fellow being, let me do it now, and not deter or neglect it, as I shall not pass this way again.
William Penn

Introduction

During my sophomore year in college I embarked upon a quest for inner peace. I yearned for relief from a persistent lack of purpose and meaning in my life. I began to study various philosophies and religions, hoping I would discover within them that elusive inner peace I sought. One evening, I was talking with a rabbi about my struggle to understand and experience faith. He told me not to worry about faith, that it didn't matter what I believed. "What matters," he said, "is how you live and what you do." These words eventually led me toward my life's work and to a realization of what inner peace is all about.

I stopped questing for inner peace, but not because I had "found" it. Rather, I realized that inner peace is not a thing to find; it follows inevitably from what we do. When we act peacefully, living with compassion and respect for everyone—people, animals, and the earth—we experience greater inner peace. Moreover, we help bring peace to our world.

This book is based on a very simple premise: *when we do the most good and the least harm through our daily choices, our acts of citizenship, our communities, our work, our volunteerism, and our interactions, we create inner and outer peace.* I call this way of living "MOGO," short for "most good," and it has become the guiding principle of my life.

The MOGO principle is simple in theory, but it asks much of us. It requires a willingness to learn new information so that we might continually reexamine our lives with the greatest good in mind and commit to conscious and deliberate choice-making for the benefit of all. Doing so calls upon us to live with integrity, courage, wisdom, perseverance, and compassion. While at first glance this might seem quite challenging, embracing the MOGO principle is deeply rewarding. It puts us on a lifelong journey that helps us realize peace within ourselves as well as create a peaceful world.

I realize that it can be very hard to imagine a peaceful world given the state of things: the horror of war, poverty, genocide, and human oppressions; the escalating degradation of the ecosystems on which all life depends; and the terrible cruelty that is perpetrated institutionally on animals. Yet we humans have faced seemingly insurmountable problems in the past, and we've triumphed many times. Apartheid in South Africa was eliminated. Mahatma Gandhi showed us that nonviolent resistance can topple an empire; and women gained the right to vote in democracies across the globe. Many people could not have imagined the end to many injustices prior to their demise. And, although humanity's cruelties and failures persist, our positive achievements are enormous and unstoppable. These positive achievements have happened because individuals like you have chosen to make a difference.

Some may be pessimistic that MOGO living can truly change intractable problems and create a peaceful, humane, and healthy world. Yet the MOGO principle is not just for the optimistic. Walking the MOGO path is joyful and meaningful in and of itself, and inevitably restores our hope as we, and others who share our vision, persevere and create healthier lives and a healthier world. As former Czech Republic president, Vaclav Havel, has written: "I feel a responsibility to work toward the things I consider good and right. I don't know whether I'll be able to change certain things for the better, or not at all. Both outcomes are possible. There is only one thing I will not concede: that it might be meaningless to strive in a good cause."[1]

• • •

---

1. Vaclav Havel, *Summer Meditations* (New York: Vintage, 1993), 17.

MOGO is not only the guiding principle of my life, it is also the foundation of my work as a humane educator—a teacher who fosters respect and compassion for all, and helps people become problem solvers and changemakers for a better world.

Since 1985, I have been teaching both youth and adults about what is happening on our planet to people, animals, and the environment, and I have been offering them the MOGO principle as a way to make their lives more positive, healthy, and helpful. After several years offering humane education classes and courses, I realized that we needed an education revolution in which all teachers became humane educators by incorporating relevant information about living sustainably, peaceably, and humanely into their existing curricula, and all schools included humane education as a subject.

I cofounded the Institute for Humane Education (IHE) in 1996 to help realize this ideal, and IHE has been training people to be humane educators and providing humane education programs ever since. We offer the first Master of Education degree focused on humane education in the United States, a Humane Education Certificate Program (HECP), and MOGO and humane education workshops and courses. People from all over the world have enrolled in our programs and workshops to learn how to be effective and inspiring humane educators and advocates for a better world, as well as to learn how to live their lives more deeply aligned with their values.

I have written this book as a humane educator who wants *everyone* to adopt the MOGO principle, both for themselves, and for the sake of the planet and all who share it. If you have picked it up because your search is primarily personal, you will discover that the path toward your own inner peace and health is the same path that will help others. It is, quite simply, much easier to be at peace with yourself if you actively pursue a MOGO life because your actions will be aligned with your values. When we feel the most conflicted inside and the most ill at ease, it is usually because we are not living with integrity; that is, not living according to what we know in our hearts and minds to be most good. Living with MOGO as a guiding principle opens us to growth, joy, renewed and renewing energy, and many and varied opportunities in life, work, and relationships.

If you have picked up *Most Good, Least Harm* because you want to help improve this world we live in, you will find many suggestions and ideas in the chapters that follow, and you may also discover that following this path significantly improves your own life. If you have ever thought that the search for inner peace was a navel-gazing retreat from the world, you will find the opposite prescription here. MOGO calls for active service and engagement.

• • •

Although my rabbi friend gave me an important piece of wisdom when he told me not to worry about what I believed, but rather about how I lived and what I did, I have come to recognize that our beliefs are quite important. What we believe largely precedes and underlies how we act.

What I have come to believe and what I hope you will also come to believe is this: *it matters that each of us chooses to lead a MOGO life to the best of our ability*. I have faith that if we each decide to live our lives based on this principle, we will not only discover greater inner peace, but we will also help bring about a genuinely peaceful and humane world.

I don't pretend to know the perfect MOGO path, let alone live it perfectly. I know that you and I will differ in our choices on this path. I know that I have as much to learn from you as I hope you have to learn from me. What matters is that we commit to the path, however we each come to understand it.

Imagine if people everywhere were committed to MOGO living. Imagine if socially responsible, humane, and environmentally sustainable companies and institutions became the norm. Imagine if governments stopped subsidizing corporations and systems that pollute and destroy, and instead supported initiatives to create sustainable, clean energies and technologies. Imagine if we promised each other and ourselves that we would solve the problems we've created and improve all of our lives in the process. Imagine the world we would create. Imagine the joy and inner peace we would experience.

We are already on the way to creating such a world. The question is, will we succeed?

The answer begins with each of us, which means it begins with you and me.

PART 1
LOOKING INWARD

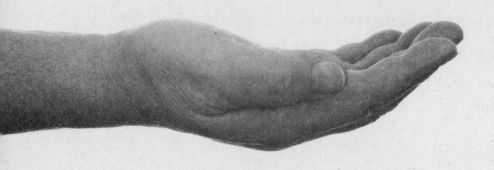

This is not a how-to book with prescribed choices for doing the most good and the least harm. It is, instead, a call to define for yourself your deepest values and to live accordingly, and this call is followed by practical information and guidelines that will help you achieve this goal. Part I offers you keys for discovering not only what is most important to you, but also what will help you traverse the MOGO path in a way that it is as healthy, joyful, and positive for you as it is for all whom your choices affect. By looking inward, you will lay the groundwork for a life that consistently does the most good and the least harm.

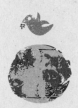

1. The Most Good, Least Harm (MOGO) Principle in Practice

As I wrote in the introduction, I am a humane educator. Humane education examines the challenges facing our planet—from human oppression, to environmental degradation, to animal cruelty, to escalating materialism—and invites people to live intentional, examined, and meaningful lives that solve the problems we face. Humane education includes four elements:

1. **Providing accurate information** about the issues of our time so that people have the information they need to confront challenges
2. **Fostering the 3 Cs: Curiosity, Creativity, and Critical thinking**, so that people have the skills to meet challenges
3. **Instilling the 3 Rs: Reverence, Respect, and Responsibility**, so that people have the motivation to face challenges
4. **Offering positive choices and tools for problem solving**, so that people are empowered to make healthy decisions for themselves and the world, and solve challenges

These are the elements I use as a humane educator, and I have incorporated them into this book so that you, too, will have the knowledge, tools, and desire to make MOGO choices. But as the reader, you will first need an element for yourself, the fifth element: *to actively and consciously cultivate what I call the* **3 Is***:* ***Inquiry, Introspection, and Integrity***.

Inquiry

In order to align your life choices with your values, you will need to inquire about the effects of your actions (and inactions) on yourself and others. Although we are always stumbling upon knowledge that shifts our choices and life direction, bringing conscious inquiry to life means that we continually ask questions that lead us to the information we need to make thoughtful decisions. Asking questions is liberating because we develop greater understanding and discover more choices with our new knowledge.

Introspection

As you ask questions and gather information, if you are to make meaningful changes, you will need to introspect—to look inward and see where the confluence of new knowledge and your life choices lies. It is likely you will periodically feel some conflict between your habits, desires, and the truth of what you have learned, but this is why a commitment to introspection is so important. When we dive below our surface desires and habits, we are able to discover our deepest visions, dreams, and commitments, which can also be quite liberating.

Integrity

As you open your heart and mind to inquiry, as you acquire the information you need to make informed and conscious decisions, and as you introspect, you are then called upon to *act* in accordance with your new knowledge and your deepest values. This is integrity, and it brings with it inner peace.

• • •

Together, these 3 *I*s help you to bring your dreams and hopes for a healthier and more joyful life—and a better world—to fruition. They make MOGO living possible by informing your everyday decisions, as well as your career, relationships, political involvement, volunteer work, recreation, and all of the ways in which you participate in creating positive change.

So far, this is all rather theoretical, so I'm going to explain how MOGO works in practice. When I teach, my students learn how to analyze products, structures, and systems, and they come to realize that there is much that is harmful in our world. In age-appropriate ways, I teach them about persistent and escalating problems and abuses behind many products, foods, clothing, and recreational options in their lives. But then, as they learn to effectively use their critical and creative thinking capacities toward imagining solutions, they begin to envision healthy and humane products, and better and more sustainable structures and systems. They discover that they have the ability to make a positive difference. Then they often make personal choices to divest themselves of those things that cause suffering and harm, as well as become change agents in an effort to bring about a better world.

In one of the activities we do, students analyze and discuss different behaviors and products, and answer the question, "Which does the most good and the least harm?" Students might compare riding a bicycle to using public transportation, driving a highly fuel-efficient car to driving a large SUV; or they might contrast a fast food hamburger to a hamburger made from grass-fed cows to an organic veggie burger. (See page 106 for more information about fast food.) They might examine the effects of a cotton T-shirt produced in an overseas sweatshop, to a cotton T-shirt produced closer to home, to an organic cotton T-shirt, to a secondhand T-shirt from a local thrift shop. (See page 32 for more on cotton T-shirts.) They might consider spending $3 a day on sodas or junk food from vending machines, versus $3 a day on healthy snacks. Or they may also consider bringing food from home and donating a percentage of their spending money to help others. There is always plenty to discuss and debate, and much to take into consideration when accounting for the effects of a choice on oneself, other people, animals, and ecosystems.

By also examining systems that perpetuate problems, these students discover that systems can change, and that their voice and involvement can make a difference. For example, they might learn about corporate charters that give corporations the rights of citizens without the concomitant responsibilities, and then learn about efforts to modify corporate charters so that companies can still pursue profits without harming the environment, people, or animals. (Please see page 100 for more information on such efforts.) Thus, not only do they become aware of the impact of their own personal choices on food, products, entertainment, and transportation, but they also learn about the power they have as citizens and members of the work and volunteer force.

As people learn to think in these ways, they generally come to discover that the MOGO principle can have far-reaching and very profound effects if put into practice by large numbers of people. Although there are rarely perfect answers to complex problems, there can be a perfectly simple principle for making choices—the MOGO principle.

As straightforward as the MOGO principle is, carrying it out in our daily lives can sometimes seem complex. Periodically, we discover a conflict between what feels best for us personally and what is likely best for other people, or what we think is best for a whole ecosystem and what might be best for individual animals, or what appears best for a specific group of people and what seems best for the environment, and so on. There will be many times when none of the individual choices within your view are ideal, and you may feel that the effort to consistently make MOGO choices is either irrelevant or too arduous.

For example, I'm typing this book on my laptop and I cannot imagine how I could do my work without this amazing machine. Yet computers are currently filled with metals that are mined in a destructive and highly polluting manner, and their components are often produced in factories where laborers suffer health problems from working with the toxic chemicals involved in computer production (and who also frequently endure sweatshop conditions). Additionally, since the "lives" of computers are so brief, these toxins wind up causing significant pollution if we discard them in landfills or incinerators.

As someone committed to living a MOGO life, what am I supposed to do with this conflict between my ethical goals and my practical need for a computer? How can I help solve the problems associated with computer use even as I rely on a computer? And, since computers represent only one example of products that come with problems, how can I address such challenges wherever and whenever they appear? What's the MOGO answer?

First, we can use the 3 *Is*, while recognizing that we may not always have perfect solutions in place right now. We can learn about the effects of our choices (bring our inquiry), figure out MOGO choices taking everything we've learned into consideration (introspect), and make MOGO choices to the extent we can (live with integrity). If ideal solutions and choices aren't available, then we can employ what I call the **3 *Vs***—our **Voice**, our **Vote**, and our monetary **Veto**—to transform systems, structures, businesses, and governments so that they, too, do the most good and the least harm.

In the case of my computer, I can educate people about the problems inherent in current computer production; support those working to create clean electronics and ensure that computer components are recycled safely; and engage in the democratic process to promote fair and safe labor standards worldwide. When I use my voice or money in favor of solutions, and vote for legislators who share my commitment to restorative, sustainable, and humane technologies, I help bring about positive change.

The MOGO principle can—and must—become the ethic that guides governments, institutions, and corporations, not just individuals. There are too many systems in place that we cannot change simply through our personal choices (such as toxins in electronics). Our world needs a revolution of values in which the MOGO principle takes root deeply and inexorably, so that we change structures that are myopic and dangerous into ones that are visionary and safe. But this won't happen unless individuals like you commit to playing a role in such a transformation. If each of us does this, we will not have to decide between our ethics and the available products and systems in place to meet our future needs. Collectively we will have resolved such problems as toxins in electronics.

Down the road, I believe we will see clothes, personal care products, transportation, appliances, food, electronics, and much more produced without destruction to the environment, without the exploitation of laborers, without cruelty to animals, without the production of toxins, without disposal systems that result in pollution, and with renewable and clean fuels. At the same time, more of us will discover that rampant consumerism is not satisfying or sustainable anyway, and we will begin to find greater joy through healthy interactions with each other and the natural world, only choosing products to meet our needs and strongest desires, and not to satisfy every whim or fill internal emptiness with stuff.

The evolution toward such a world is both essential and possible. With shifts in the way we think and changes in educational, political, and corporate priorities, we can make the world evolve. But these changes won't come about without a group of people working to make this vision real. And this group will not come from one political party, one socioeconomic bracket, one religion, one age group, or one nation. It will form from people across all spectrums of life who want future generations to thrive and survive; who cannot bear the rapid extinction of species or the despoiling of our earth; who believe in justice and equality; who long for meaning and joy; and who are committed to doing the most good and the least harm. It will be both our individual lives and the collective movement growing from our combined efforts that will transform the world into one in which our choices are healthy, sustainable, peaceful, and just.

MOGO is a way of assessing choices; it is not a cookie-cutter formula. What is most good and least harmful will often be somewhat subjective and need to take into account many variables. It will be up to you to decide for yourself. The challenge is to do so with commitment, honesty, and integrity.

•••

You may wonder whether bringing the 3 *I*s to every choice and employing the 3 *V*s wherever entrenched problems exist might turn your life into a state of constant analysis and weigh you down with a moral nag. That hardly sounds like it would bring much inner peace. The truth is that you *could* become caught up with every detail of your life and drive yourself crazy, but that would definitely not be MOGO.

Instead, you can bring open-minded effort and commitment to examined choice-making to the decisions in your life—what you buy, eat, and wear; what you do for work; how you participate in creating positive change; how you take care of yourself—all without berating yourself for being imperfect. If we ask what will do the most good and the least harm (or sometimes, what will simply do more good and less harm) in relation to these and other choices, we set the stage for far-reaching positive effects rather than for personal purity.

Ultimately, when we choose the MOGO principle we will:

- Have a simple, helpful, and meaningful guide for every choice, conflict, issue, and life decision we will ever face
- Cultivate our own wisdom and kindness
- Increase our freedom from others' imperatives, whether these come from advertisers, social norms, the media, or individual people telling us what we should or shouldn't do
- Improve our own lives without unknowingly or unjustifiably harming others or the environment to do so
- Stay honest
- Remain humble, open, and nonjudgmental
- Balance strong concerns with level-headed choice-making
- Develop our self-discipline and equanimity
- Free ourselves from the specter of guilt, indignity, or shame caused by unreflective, inhumane, or rash decision-making
- Be liberated from the oppressive pursuit of perfection

Seen in this way, what at first might seem like work turns out instead to be an opportunity for a better life for ourselves, everyone our lives affect, as well as our environment.

We're all aware of the Golden Rule to "do unto others as we would have them do unto us." Whether phrased in the positive or negative (don't do unto others what we wouldn't want done unto us), this "rule" is integral to every major religion and has been prescribed by philosophers over millennia. In the King James version of the New Testament, this rule reads: "And as ye would that men should do to you, do ye also to them likewise." Buddhist scripture asks: "A state that is not pleasing or delightful to me, how could I inflict that upon another?" In Islam: "None of you truly believes until he wishes for his brother what he wishes for himself." In Judaism: "What is hateful to you, do not do to your fellow man. This is the law: all the rest is commentary." Plato wrote, "May I do to others as I would that they should do unto me." And the British Humanist Society left it simply as, "Don't do things you wouldn't want to have done to you."[1] There are many more versions from Hinduism, Taoism, Sufism, Jainism, Confucianism, Zoroastrianism, and numerous spiritual traditions among indigenous peoples across the globe, but I think I've belabored the point enough. The Golden Rule is a foundational principle among humans everywhere.

But now our complex world requires a new Golden Rule, one that enables us to put into practice the original Golden Rule universally. In a world in which our clothes, food, transportation, fuel, products, and homes come to us through a web of connections that extend around the planet, we need a principle to guide us so that we actually can do to others, no matter how geographically distant, as we would have them do to us, and refrain from doing to others that which is abhorrent to us. Most good, least harm is that principle. MOGO calls upon us to raise our awareness and connect the dots between ourselves and others whom our life impacts so that we can make sure that we are not being abusive or oppressive, and instead are increasing joy, health, and equality for everyone.

---

1. See http://www.religioustolerance.org/reciproc.htm.

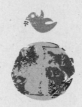

2. Seven Keys to MOGO

It is easy enough to say that if we do the most good and the least harm, our lives will improve and our positive impact on the world will increase significantly, but to actually live the MOGO principle, it helps to use the following seven keys:

Key 1—Live Your Epitaph
Key 2—Pursue Joy through Service
Key 3—Make Connections and Self-Reflect
Key 4—Model Your Message and Work for Change
Key 5—Find and Create Community
Key 6—Take Responsibility
Key 7—Strive for Balance

There are likely other keys that you will discover on your path, but by using these seven as a guide, you'll have solid, helpful tools to put MOGO into practice; achieve your goals; stay balanced, healthy, and peaceful; and contribute to a better world.

Key 1—Live Your Epitaph

Imagine that you are very old, approaching the end of your life. You're sitting on a park bench, remembering a time when we humans killed and exploited one another, despoiled our planet, abused animals, and allowed our neighbors around the world to go hungry. While you are breathing the clean air on our now safe and healthy planet, and thinking about that dark period from your past, a child comes up to you. The child has learned about that dangerous, destructive time in history class and asks you, "What role did you play in helping to bring about the world we have today?"

What will you tell this child?

Please consider this question for a few minutes before you continue reading.

• • •

Each day of your life you are part of creating this child's future. When you do the most good and the least harm, you set in motion the forces that will make a healthy and humane future possible for generations of all species on earth. Your response to the question above is a way of answering, "What would I like my epitaph to be?" If you can imagine an epitaph that feels worthy of your life, then you can choose to live it—to embody and realize your goals and values more consciously and effectively.

To lead a MOGO life, each of us must determine our deepest values and live accordingly. Each of us would write a different epitaph, and each of us would interpret our vision of a MOGO life in a unique manner. I have three friends and colleagues, Melissa Feldman, Khalif Williams, and Kim Korona, whom I admire immensely because they endeavor to live their epitaph each day of their lives. They are vibrant, honest, generous, and an inspiration to me, each in their own way. And they also live very differently from one another, which reminds us that there is no best epitaph to live, and no one model for a MOGO life. As you read about them in the next few pages, notice the variety of ways in which they have interpreted MOGO living and how they are manifesting their desired epitaph.

Melissa Feldman

Melissa was raised in an upper middle class home by compassionate, environmentally conscious, and loving parents who rescued stray dogs and cats, and recycled before it was common-place to do so. She, too, was deeply empathetic and caring, find-ing herself, for example, refusing to go to the zoo as a young child because it depressed her to see the big cats pacing back and forth in their small cages.

When she grew up to be a tall, slender, and beautiful young woman, she discovered opportunities in the fashion industry. Attracted by the glamour, salary, and travel, and the chance to mix with the rich and famous, Melissa first became a model and then was hired to work for a renowned designer.

Melissa found herself living in two worlds: the world of her deepest values and the world of her career, which demanded cer-tain behaviors and attitudes. She complied with the requirements of her job, building a callous shell that allowed her to reject the hopeful teenage girls who came to audition for modeling oppor-tunities—without even addressing them by name. She began to choose friends based on their appearance, not their personalities or their character.

The growing conflict between Melissa's deepest values and the requirements of her job became difficult to reconcile. One day, she was asked to create a fashion show for fur coats. She strug-gled to justify a fashion show that caused such unnecessary cru-elty and suffering to animals, but she couldn't do it. The next day she quit her lucrative job and left her high-status career. She took a low-paying job at a humane society and later went back to school to earn a Master of Education degree.

Since then, Melissa has been giving others the critical thinking tools to resist advertising's influence. Through her innovative pro-gram, Circle of Compassion, she tells young people her story, teaches them to become adept at analyzing the messages that come their way through the media, and explains what happens in the sweatshops behind brand names and to the animals killed for fur. She's taken her enormous creativity and style and designed brilliant activities that people of all ages love. She parades around a classroom in the huge eyeglasses she wore in the 1970s and asks her students what they think of them before replacing them with her current pair and asks them again. She carries a little blue

Tiffany bag and invites students to shout out their assumptions about her based on her bag, then follows with a Victoria's Secret shopping bag, and then a Wal-Mart plastic bag. She asks them if they can recognize a brand simply by its color, and pulls out a navy blue bag, folded in such a way that the company's name is hidden. Her students quickly shout out the Gap. By the time she's done, no student can listen to a jingle without realizing how thoroughly media messages have invaded their ideas and even their beliefs, all without their consent, their effort, or even their awareness. All leave with new skills for identifying their values and living accordingly. All begin to reassess what matters most to them.

Melissa is fifty years old, and lives simply and happily these days in a two-bedroom apartment in Boston that she shares with a roommate. She is honest, funny, warm, and kind. She never speaks poorly of others and is one of the most trustworthy people I have ever known. She still enjoys shopping and she dresses very fashionably, but now she buys her clothes based on her values. She fosters rescued greyhounds, makes handmade gifts for those she loves, and makes friends based on their personalities, not their looks. And she teaches the next generation how to avoid the mistakes she made when she was young.

When I asked Melissa to tell me how she interprets the MOGO principle, she answered this way:

> MOGO starts with me. As they say on the airlines, in case of a loss of oxygen, put on your oxygen mask first and then help your kids put on their masks. I believe that I deserve to have a good and happy life, even though others are suffering. This was a hard concept for me to understand years ago. At the same time, one of the cardinal philosophies of my life comes from Helen Keller, who said, "I am only one, but still I am one. I cannot do everything, but still I can do something. I will not refuse to do the something I can do." So I start with myself, but I don't end there.
>
> My major efforts to create positive change include being a humane educator and living a life that models my mes-

sage. I also write letters and make phone calls. I had a volunteer job that I really liked, working every Saturday for several years for a nonprofit that provided low-income women with interview suits. That was a great match for me.

I like to help people directly, but I don't give money to every person I see who is homeless. My rule is [that] I buy the local homeless paper, *Spare Change*, whenever I see it. Sometimes that means I buy a paper every day. I also give to people who are homeless if they have a child or an animal. These are arbitrary rules that have more to do with me than with the actual needs of others, but these rules help me get through the day.

It might seem like Melissa faces no conflicts in her choice-making or that she always knows how to follow the MOGO principle, but she does experience challenges.

It's hard at times to do what I think is best. For example, I'm still using disposable cameras. I've convinced myself that I will borrow someone's digital camera if I really need to take a lot of pictures, or I'll just break down and buy one, or I'll wait for someone I know to get a new one and give me their old one. As a result of my wishful thinking but total inaction, none of these things have happened, and I'm still using film and disposable cameras. The thought of researching which camera to buy and which company has the best track record, or the least bad as far as pollution and employee treatment go, is daunting. So I've chosen the nonchoice, and every time I buy one more disposable camera, I say to myself that this will be the last one. [Several months after Melissa told me this, a friend gave her a used digital camera, so she is now no longer using disposable cameras.]

Another obstacle I face is composting. I live in an apartment in Boston, but I still could do it. My partner lives in the wilds of New Hampshire, and I could simply bring my food scraps to his place every weekend or connect with someone who has one of the city gardening spots in my neighborhood. And yet, I haven't so far.

Two other issues that have been on my mind are the prisoners at Guantánamo Bay and women's rights, particularly in Africa. I have done nothing but talk about these issues. I have not written one letter, made one phone call, or donated one dollar to help.

I guess the way I think about these challenges is this: I do the best I can for today. I'm comfortable being uncomfortable with some of my choices. I know that I'm moving in a direction of greater compassion, and overall I'm throwing more positive energy out into the universe than negative. I don't want to punish myself into composting. I know I will get to it and to many other things on a long list. I don't think putting negative, shaming, berating energy into the world will help make it better.

At a certain point, I will become uncomfortable with some of my less-than-MOGO choices and make compassionate changes. For example, I already have taken steps to minimize electricity for heating and cooling. In my top floor apartment, we now make it through winters in Boston without ever putting on the heat. I've come up with some tricks in the summer to minimize air conditioning, and soon I will have to replace my AC unit with a newer unit that is more energy efficient. But still, I do want AC. I think I ultimately will feel good about the choice, knowing I'm making an environmentally unfriendly choice in the most friendly way possible. I can live with that.

To refer back to another one of my examples, I guess my concern about women in Africa had been ruminating somewhere inside me despite my outward inaction. As a result and quite by accident, I have a new friend, Barbara, a refugee from Liberia. We met on the subway when Barbara asked me for directions. Out of that accidental moment, a friendship has developed unlike any other friendship I've ever had before. Barbara has been an unexpected gift in my life and as a result of being open to this chance encounter, I not only have more community, love, and friends in my life, but I have also been able to be of service to Barbara and her family in small ways.

What does Melissa want her epitaph to say?

"Melissa did some good and had some fun along the way."

I love Melissa. I love her acceptance of herself and others, her nonjudgmental attitude, and her perseverance. She is a role model of all these qualities for me. When I am busy judging, I think of Melissa, and I remind myself that the way to manifest MOGO includes acceptance and a positive attitude.

Khalif Williams

I met Khalif Williams in 2001 when he attended a workshop I led at Haverford College near Philadelphia. He was so engaged, eager to learn and share, and full of enthusiasm and vision. I have led many workshops and met many people in my work, but Khalif so stood out that when I ran into him six months later at a conference, not only did I recognize him, I also remembered his name—a rarity for me. Khalif joined our staff at the Institute for Humane Education in 2002 and became our executive director a couple of years later.

Khalif, who is thirty-five, and his wife, Amy Bramblett, have two children and live in a beautiful five-hundred-eighty-square-foot house that Khalif designed and built himself, with some help from friends in the community. Khalif and Amy had bought a small piece of land, cleared it themselves, and did everything possible to make the house ecologically friendly. They live without electricity. Almost all the windows and doors have been salvaged, as have most of the interior wood paneling and stairs. They heat with wood, mostly waste softwood found locally or cut right from their property, refrigerate with block ice (purchased or home-made, depending on the season), and light with oil lamps. They plan to install solar electricity eventually, which will eliminate their lamp oil consumption and ice purchasing in the summer. As Khalif says:

The old joke about running water applies to us: when we want water, we just run outside to the pump and get some. We keep a fifty-five-gallon rain barrel full of water in the loft for washing which is gravity fed to the kitchen sink. Bathing, at least for now, takes place in the middle of the living room floor in an eighty-gallon livestock watering trough, Japanese style. Our baths usually take less than three gallons of water, and we get just as clean as when we lived with a full shower. We've actually come to prefer this way of bathing. I'm currently in the process of building a bathhouse where we'll bathe and take saunas. We also use a composting toilet, producing "humanure."

Khalif's family eats a lot of seasonal, local food, as much organic as they can afford, and a little packaged food from time to time. They use only biodegradable cleaning products and very little of them. They purchase very few new items and prefer secondhand for almost everything. They own very few things that they don't actually need.

Khalif's lifestyle is quite different, not only from Melissa's but also from most people in industrialized countries. It's possible that his lifestyle sounds extreme to you, but the vast majority of the people in the world live more like Khalif than like the typical reader of this book. Khalif didn't grow up living the way he lives now, however. He was raised in northwestern Pennsylvania, and his family had as many material possessions as the average family in the United States. He watched lots of television, and no one in his family paid attention to the impact of the food they ate or the products they used.

Khalif has chosen a different way of life because it is important to him to minimize the harm he causes to others and the environment. The more equilibrium he can create in his life—giving back as much as he takes, creating little waste and actually using what others call waste, increasing the positive impact he has on the world—the better he feels. As he says, "It gives me great satisfaction. I don't think I've reached any sort of perfection. Far from it. I'm a million miles away, but trying is very fun."

Khalif goes on to say, "There is nothing difficult or special about living as I do. It seems much more difficult to do anything else. Others may experience greater convenience living a more typical life, but that's only because the conveniences are paid for further upstream."

What would Khalif want his epitaph to say?

"Khalif Williams gave all he had, took only what he needed, and would have loved you with all his heart."

A few final words about Khalif: he and his family don't live an isolated life in the woods. They have created an extraordinary community. This community helped him build his home, and he helps everyone else in the community, too. They've established a bimonthly work party in which about a dozen families gather every other Sunday at someone's house to join together and work on projects. They bring food to share; the children in the community play together (and help as they are able); and when the work is done, everyone enjoys a meal and makes music. If ever there were a richer, more meaningful, more joyful life, I've yet to witness it.

Kim Korona

I met Kim Korona when she enrolled in our Master of Education program. Just out of college, Kim was young in age but wise beyond her years. I took to calling her the kindest person I know. I still introduce her this way—much to her dismay, as Kim is also one of the most humble people I've ever met. I suppose that's not very MOGO of me, and I should probably stop introducing her like this, but Kim is simply my MOGO role model for kindness.

Kim is now twenty-seven years old and a humane educator at HEART, where she teaches humane education classes to middle and high school students throughout New York City. She has also created her own group, Chrysalis, whose mission is to bring environmental preservation, human rights, animal protection, and media literacy organizations together to promote holistic collaboration and education.

Kim grew up in a lower middle class family in Detroit, Michigan, but as a child she did not think about her family's socioeconomic status. Her parents provided for all of her and her sister's needs, working opposite shifts so that one of them was always home, a sacrifice she has only recently begun to appreciate. Growing up, her family lived in a racially diverse neighborhood, until slowly all of the white people began to move away, including her family. This move significantly affected Kim, making her question segregated communities and appreciate diversity. Once she was an adult, she chose to move back into a racially and ethnically diverse neighborhood in Detroit's inner city before her move to New York.

For Kim, living with the MOGO principle in mind simply means examining her choices. She considers how a choice will affect her, those around her, other people in the world, other species, and the planet itself. She admits that it can be difficult to really know how her decisions affect everyone else and the environment, especially if she has limited information; and sometimes she finds it hard to choose what is in the best interest of someone or something that she cannot see, especially when it appears that it will give a lot of happiness to someone who is in need right in front of her. For example, Kim chooses to eat a complete vegetarian (vegan) diet because she believes that it does the most good and the least harm to the environment, to animals, and to her health. When she was in Mexico, volunteering at El Centro del Esperanza (The Center for Hope), she was asked to make ham sandwiches for the children. When she looked at the hungry children, there was no way she was going to say no; that didn't seem MOGO to her at all. She wished she had bought food for them that didn't cause suffering to animals, but she hadn't, so she chose to make the sandwiches for the children. When she came home, however, she decided to find the MOGO answer to this predicament. She began to provide organic, vegan soups for people who were homeless in Detroit. This way she was able to help people who were hungry without compromising her commitment to also help animals and the environment.

Kim has been involved in a variety of community groups and she always aims to practice her volunteerism with the MOGO ethic. She and her boyfriend, Tom, volunteered at an organic community garden in Detroit. Tom revitalized the garden as a way to help a young man find some direction in his life. The garden has since served as a catalyst for Kim's work teaching values of cooperation, dedication, and patience. Together they have used the garden as a center for education programs focusing on the treatment of others; concerns with factory farming; and the value of local, organic, healthy food. In her activism, Kim acts with this adage in mind: People will forget most of what you say and some of what you did, but they will never forget how you made them feel. It should come as no surprise that Kim makes everyone around her feel welcomed, accepted, and loved.

I asked Kim how it feels to live her life with the MOGO principle in mind.

It is a life that is full of joy in which I feel a wholeness in my spirit. There are certainly challenges, because, in being so aware when I do something that I know is not the MOGO choice, I sometimes feel sadness and guilt. I question myself and wonder why I made the choice I made. But then I thoughtfully consider the choice and work to make a more humane one the next time. The wonderful part about MOGO is that it is not about living a perfect life, which is not possible to do. Instead, it is about being mindful of my choices, because I feel the interconnectedness of the world. I think that I am helping to create a more peaceful world with the choices I make, and that brings me great joy.

There are so many problems in the world, and I used to wonder what the most important work was. Then I realized I needed to ask myself a different question. Based on who I am, how can I best serve the world? We must consider our best talents and strongest interests, and discover how we can put the two together.

Some people may wonder if a MOGO life is difficult because of the sacrifices they might be called upon to make, but I find that as one realizes the positive impact one is having on the world, nothing feels like a sacrifice. Life feels rejuvenating because it isn't superficial, and our actions become much more intentional and purposeful. Most people are looking for meaning and purpose. A MOGO life gives us this.

As for Kim's epitaph, here's how she'd like it to read:

"Kimberly Korona believed that if we wanted to, we could create a humane world for all people, all species, and the entire planet, and so she strived to contribute her part in creating such a world and to inspire others to do the same."

• • •

Melissa, Khalif, and Kim are different ages, are from different ethnicities and races, live in different kinds of communities, are from different socioeconomic strata, and have chosen different kinds of families, but what they have in common is an abiding commitment to deeply embody their values and live worthwhile and generously engaged lives; they live their epitaphs. They also have this in common: none is a dour do-gooder, and none feels deprived.

There is no way to tally up someone's life to determine who has done the most good and the least harm, although many will try to tell others exactly which choices are best. I'm wary of anyone, be they a religious leader, politician, or teacher, who asks you to follow their one and only way, the "perfectly true" path. I'm equally wary of moral relativists who profess that good and bad are always qualified. And I'm most disturbed by those who say that our choices don't matter. As Melissa, Khalif, and Kim would tell you, they matter enormously.

The choices you make in your life matter to you; to your family, friends, and neighbors; and to all those whom your life impacts. They matter to the people who work in mines to extract the minerals you rely upon; who grow, pick, and slaughter what you eat; who make your clothes; who put together your electronics; and so much more. They matter to the animals whose habitats are being destroyed and whose lives are made miserable for a dietary preference or a product choice. It matters to the overall health and well-being of the planet, and the ecosystems that connect us all when your choices cause destruction, create excessive carbon in the atmosphere, pollute, or cause unsustainable resource depletion and waste. Thus, it matters that you identify your deepest values, consider your epitaph, and live accordingly.

Living your epitaph may also be the most important ingredient for inner peace and serenity. When you actively align your choices with your life's purpose and goals, you live more honestly, courageously, and with greater integrity, and these virtues bring with them a powerful kind of freedom. While no one lives their epitaph perfectly, the more we endeavor to do this, and the more frequently we make choices that are mindful and in accordance with our vision for our life, the more we discover peace within ourselves and the greater our positive impact on the world.

There is a story about a Cherokee grandfather who is teaching his grandson about life. He says to his grandson, "A fight is going on inside me. It is a terrible fight between two wolves. One is evil; he is anger, envy, greed, arrogance, self-pity, resentment, and superiority. The other is good; he is joy, peace, love, hope, humility, generosity, and compassion. This same fight is going on inside you, and inside every other person, too."

The grandson thinks about this for a minute and then asks his grandfather, "Which wolf will win?"

The old Cherokee simply replies, "The one we feed."

Below, you will find a list of qualities that I've gathered from groups of people who have answered the question, "What are the best qualities of human beings?" As you read this list, consider which qualities you want to feed. Which inspire you to grow, change, and develop in new ways? Which feel essential to your epitaph? Try reading each one silently and slowly; notice if the quality speaks to you and invites you to listen more deeply:

Compassion, Kindness, Creativity, Trustworthiness, Humility, Perseverance, Wisdom, Gratitude, Tolerance, Altruism, Patience, Forgiveness, Curiosity, Resilience, Respect, Self-discipline,

Gentleness, Tenderness, Attentiveness, Commitment, Initiative, Willingness to be Different, Willingness to Choose and Change, Mindfulness, Expressiveness, Courtesy, Resourcefulness, Flexibility, Adaptability, Optimism, Sensitivity, Strength, Graciousness, Loyalty, Hopefulness, Mercy, Vibrancy, Peacefulness, Self-awareness, Ingenuity, Willingness to Rise Above Circumstances, Equanimity, Helpfulness, Humor.

By considering the epitaph you want, you give yourself the greatest opportunity to actually live your values and practice MOGO. This first key to MOGO begins a process from which the rest will follow with clarity and purpose. (When you complete the **MOGO Questionnaire and Action Plan** in part III, you'll have the opportunity to put into words your desired epitaph.)

Key 2—Pursue Joy through Service

When I was contemplating this key, I initially perceived it as two separate keys: (1) Pursue Joy, and (2) Be of Service. I believe that joy is a critical ingredient in a MOGO life, not only because it's most good for us as individuals to experience joy, but also because few are going to want to commit to MOGO living if it feels like drudgery and they rarely feel joyful.

I decided to conduct an unofficial survey of several hundred people asking them, "What brings you joy?" I was curious about whether pursuing joy was commonly compatible with pursuing MOGO. It's been my experience that it is, but I wanted to make sure that this was true for others. Given that MOGO living seems at first glance to demand sacrifice, I felt that, to be honest about the benefits to ourselves, I should find out if experiences of joy were potentially contrary to choosing MOGO. Maybe the things that brought people joy were the same things that unwittingly caused harm to other people, animals, and the environment.

In the responses to my survey, no one told me that a new SUV or a big house brought joy. There were no paeans to perfect, pesticide-sprayed lawns or eating *foie gras*. People wrote about being with children, loved ones, and animals, and told me about joyful experiences in nature. They also wrote about something else: over and over, they mentioned service. When I read their impassioned words about service, I realized that these two perceived keys were really one, and a beautiful one at that: pursue joy through service.

Here's what some had to say in response to the question, "What brings you joy?"

One of the most joyous things I can experience is to see many people coming together for a common, good cause.
—**Faye Harbottle, Washington, DC**

Service brings me joy. It has been the organizing principle of my adult life, informing my career decisions, and my spiritual and political beliefs. On many days, it has been what gets me out of bed in the morning. It has brought extraordinary people into my life, and has provided me with opportunities to see and do things I never could have imagined.
—**Carla Ganiel, Maine**

My joy stems from a constant realization that justice will prevail, and I'm taking part in bringing justice to the world a little bit more quickly.
—**Bruce Friedrich, Washington, DC**

Asking a homeless person what he or she would like to eat; giving them some extra cash; exchanging a sincere, heartfelt smile; then seeing that same person the following week at the same gas station market, greeting them by name and knowing what they want, and seeing their joy when I give it to them.
—**Doriane Lucia, California**

Most of the joys I experience are small ones, like eating an apple after I run, encountering an unexpected wild critter, seeing the river mirror-smooth, finding a new connection between ideas, or enjoying a conversation. I remember a range of stronger joys.... These haven't disappeared, but they are quieter nowadays.... I think I'm happier now with a steady stream of joys, all within reach, than I was earlier in life with a feast and famine of joys. I also think I'm more peaceful and more kind now, but I suspect that my allotment of joys is more an effect than a cause of this development.

—Peter Suber, Maine

The belief that doing good brings happiness is as old as history. Socrates, described in Plato's *Republic*, said, "Only those who act rightly are truly happy."[1] In his book *Field Notes on the Compassionate Life*, Marc Ian Barasch explores not only compassion and kindness but also their cousin: altruism. When reading the accounts in this book, we discover that the happiest people seem to be the ones who are most likely to help others, even going so far as to donate a kidney to a stranger. After natural disasters, when good Samaritans are interviewed regularly by the media, it is practically always the case that it is the most joyful people who open their homes, hearts, and pocketbooks to strangers.

Although I haven't met him myself, many friends and colleagues have met His Holiness the Dalai Lama, and all of them comment on a quality that the Dalai Lama possesses in abundance: joyful kindness. The author of the book, *My Religion is Kindness*, the Dalai Lama is a living example of the connection between service, peace, and compassion on the one hand, and personal joy and inner peace on the other.

Research also shows that doing good improves our lives. There are hundreds of studies that demonstrate the life-enhancing benefits of kindness and compassion. When we give of ourselves, especially if we start young, evidence indicates that we live longer, are less depressed, and are healthier and more self-realized.[2]

---

1. Quoted in Peter Singer's *Writings on an Ethical Life* (New York: Harper Perennial, 2001), 246.

2. See Stephen Post's *Why Good Things Happen to Good People* (New York: Broadway, 2008).

There was a period of time during and after college and in graduate school when I did a lot of volunteer work. I taught English to a Vietnamese refugee in South Philadelphia, helped out in a program for young adults at a mental hospital, led tours at a natural history museum, regularly visited the inmates at a women's prison, and served as a court companion to victims of rape—and other volunteer work.

But I'm no saint. I did all these activities because they served *me*. Helping others was satisfying, interesting, meaningful, and enriching. Unexpectedly (and delightfully), one of these volunteer jobs led to paid work. I wouldn't have been hired at my first full-time job as a teacher and naturalist at a wildlife rehabilitation and nature center had I not volunteered at the natural history museum and gained a referral. And that first job led to others, which led to finding my life's work as a humane educator, for which I'm very grateful. That's what can happen when we volunteer our time to help others.

It's important to find the right ways to give, though. When I get a call to bake cookies for some event at my son's school, I admit that I sometimes feel put upon. When I do agree to bake the cookies, my motivation stems more from guilt than joy in giving. This is because I'm not crazy about doing any more cooking than I already do. But ask me to lead a service at our local Unitarian Universalist Church or to volunteer to teach for a week at my son's school (tasks equivalent in time to baking enormous quantities of cookies), and I'm excited to give of my time and energy. It's crucial to find ways in which you find joy in giving so that you're not a resentful do-gooder, but instead a radiant person of service.

Some people have more money than time to give, and their generosity fuels enormously important efforts that would be paralyzed without the dollars that they supply. If you have the ability to make financial contributions to better the world, by all means give what you can monetarily. Jews are expected to give 10 percent of their income to charity, for example. For those who barely scrape by on their earnings, 10 percent might be out of reach. But for others 10 percent might be far less than they are able to give, and they may be able to increase the percentage to 20 percent or more. I know a man who donates every penny beyond what he personally needs to nonprofit, social change groups. For him, each salary increase represents the opportunity to give more.

When we contemplate the time we are given—in a year, or in a week, or even in a day—we discover that this time is our life. What do you want to do with this life? When we meditate for even a moment on this question, we may realize just how important it is to use some of our time to give of ourselves. The Prayer of St. Francis offers a reminder:

> *Lord, make me an instrument of peace.*
> *Where there is hatred, let me sow love,*
> *Where there is injury, pardon,*
> *Where there is doubt, faith,*
> *Where there is despair, hope,*
> *Where there is darkness, light,*
> *Where there is sadness, joy.*
> *O divine master, grant that I may not so much seek*
> *to be consoled, as to console,*
> *To be understood as to understand,*
> *To be loved as to love.*
> *For it is in giving that we receive,*
> *It is in pardoning that we are pardoned,*
> *And it is in dying that we are born to eternal life.*

It is in giving that we receive. We know what happens when we give to others. Life gets better for them and for us. With all this said, however, it can feel burdensome for many people to think of being of greater service to others. Many of our lives are so full of the tasks of daily living (and then collapsing at the end of each day) that giving to others may feel like the last thing we want to do, even if it would make us more joyful. If we're raising children or taking care of elderly parents, we may already feel overwhelmed in the service department. If we're full-time students with homework to do and a job on top of our studies, service might seem impossible. If we're working two jobs to make ends meet, the idea of service may seem like a luxury for the privileged and not a reality for us. Joy itself may seem out of reach, with pleasure being the grail we seek to make exhausting situations endurable.

But pleasure may not be as satisfying as we think. When we put ourselves in situations in which we are likely to experience joy, as opposed to simply pleasure, it is restoring and life-affirming. Pleasure feels nice; joy deeply and completely fills our heart and soul. Pleasure is generally time-limited and often specific to actions, such as eating good food or watching a favorite television show; joy suffuses our entire being with vitality. Pleasure can be contained within you; more often than not, joy radiates outward toward others.

There is another way that pleasure and joy diverge. Pleasure can be addictive—a hunger that's never quite sated—whereas joy does not require that we fulfill our personal desires, as its link to service demonstrates. The pursuit of pleasure can actually stand in the way of experiencing joy.

The mystic Saint Teresa of Avila wrote this about joy:

> *Her heart is full of joy with love, . . .*
> *She has renounced every selfish attachment*
> *And draws abiding joy and strength from the One within.*
> *She lives not for herself, but lives to serve the*
> *Lord of Love in all,*
> *And swims across the sea of life, breasting its*
> *rough waves joyfully.*[3]

Few are going to commit to the path of MOGO living if those on this path are not joyful and deeply alive people. But many will choose to do the most good and the least harm when they see the radiant joy embodied by people who live their lives meaningfully,

---

3. Eknath Easwaran, *God Makes the Rivers to Flow: Selections from the Sacred Literature of the World* (Tomales, CA: Nilgiri Press, 1992), 66.

generously, and with kindness and service toward others. When people witness the creativity, beauty, and positive transformations that follow your passion to help, they may be moved to emulate you, and their lives may become more joyful as well.

Practical Ideas for Joyful Service

- Volunteer where your help is needed, doing something that you enjoy.[4]
- Join a service group such as Rotary or Lions Club.[5]
- Make donations to organizations working to change oppressive and destructive systems into ones that are positive, sustainable, peaceful, and just.
- Experience joy as a side effect of kindness by trying some of the following:
  - Tell those you love what you love about them.
  - Give up something that causes harm. Mahatma Gandhi made it a practice to give up things to free himself of attachments to pleasure, and to receive the deeper experience of reverence and joy.
  - Smile at people.
  - Let others share their stories with you.
  - Give your seat on the bus or subway to someone who needs it more than you.
  - Hold doors open.
  - Let people in your lane of traffic.
- If none of the suggestions above appeal to you, that does not mean that you can't be of service. Search within. What can you offer that would bring joy to you and would be of value to others?
- See chapter 6, **Activism, Volunteerism, and Democracy**, for many more examples and suggestions.

---

4. Visit http://www.volunteermatch.org for ideas and places to volunteer in your region.

5. Visit http://www.rotary.org and http://www.lionsclub.org.

Key 3—Make Connections and Self-Reflect

What is the connection between the Gulf of Mexico dead zone (an area approximately the size of New Jersey that can no longer support life) and the fact that 22 percent of American teenagers are reportedly overweight?

This question is one that David Orr, a professor of environmental studies and politics at Oberlin College, asked students in one of his courses. As he describes it, "After an hour, they had filled the blackboard with boxes and arrows that included federal farm subsidies, U.S. tax law, chemical dependency, feedlots and megafarms, the rise of the fast food industry, declining farm communities, corporate centralization, advertising, a cheap food policy, research agendas at land-grant institutions, urban sprawl, the failure of political institutions, cheap fossil energy, and so forth."[6]

To translate: the dead zone in the Gulf of Mexico exists because the polluted Mississippi River flows into the Gulf, and the mix of agricultural runoff from industrial farms is deadly. This kind of industrial farming is part of a system that produces unhealthy, high-calorie, highly advertised food—thus the connection to overweight teens.

In order to make MOGO choices, and create a humane and sustainable world, we are going to have to become adept at making connections. Single-issue thinking and taking sides when issues are presented to us in simplistic terms will have to give way to far more nuanced research, consideration, and decision making. Fortunately, the information age in which we live provides the opportunity for understanding the connections between an ocean dead zone and overweight people; between rising cancer rates and laws that give corporations the rights of persons without the concomitant responsibility not to harm others through toxic emissions; between increasingly devastating natural disasters, and legal and economic decisions that further short-term gains over long-term safety; between corporate financing of elections and a failure to pass laws that protect diversity on the planet;

---

6. David Orr, *The Last Refuge* (Washington, D.C.: Island Press, 2005), 66.

between a growing population of poor, disenfranchised people and escalating worldwide slavery; and so on. But we won't make any of these connections unless we actively inquire and seek to find them.

Dr. Orr's question to his students provides them with the opportunity to make connections that are normally ignored in our society. We don't usually look at a single issue, such as a lifeless section of ocean or growing obesity rates, and draw a web. We generally prefer more simple cause-and-effect discussions and conclusions. But the issues of our time are complex and require research and effort to understand; and the daily choices we make, while seemingly insignificant, have hidden effects that we will never see or understand if we don't make an effort to make connections.

When I teach in schools, I often bring an item into the classroom—or invite students to pick an item of their own—and ask them to examine its true cost to themselves, other people, animals, and the environment. We'll do this more in the next chapter, **Products**, but the point here is that when we cast our gaze beyond the product itself, we begin to understand the ways in which its effects weave inextricably into others' lives, the health of ecosystems, animals, our own well-being, and the economy. As an example of making connections, let's bring our inquiry to one of the most common products in our culture—the ubiquitous cotton T-shirt.

Cotton is the world's most heavily pesticide-sprayed crop, accounting for approximately 10 percent of global pesticide use. These include highly toxic chemicals that wind up in waterways, poisoning fishes and affecting the entire food chain, including humans. The cotton that is produced in Asia is often grown, sprayed, and picked by children who are exposed to these dangerous toxins without any protective clothing or masks. Cotton is also a crop that requires significant irrigation and is highly energy-intensive in its production.

Once the cotton is harvested and woven into fabric, it is usually dyed using hazardous textile dyes. Approximately 30 percent of the dye (which does not adhere to the cotton) is carried off into the wastewater stream.

Cottonseed oil, a byproduct of the cotton industry, is used in a variety of foods, most notably in snack foods. Yet cotton is not regulated as a food crop and, as described above, is heavily sprayed with fungicides and insecticides.

More often than not, conventional T-shirts are sewn in overseas factories that are not required to follow the same labor laws as in wealthy countries. This means that in many—if not most—factories, workers, including children, may suffer from some or all of the following: they are paid less than their country's minimum wage; they work under extremely unhealthy and often dangerous conditions; they receive none of the benefits common among factory workers in richer countries; they are unable to form unions and are fired for trying to do so; and they work excessively long hours. It may be true that these sweatshop jobs are better than no jobs, but those do not have to be the only two choices. We can improve conditions for people working in harsh conditions through the 3 Vs (again, our Voice, our Vote, and our monetary Veto).

The finished T-shirts are exported, often across the globe, using significant amounts of fossil fuels in the process. They are then displayed in stores that we each travel to, usually using more fossil fuels, in order to buy them.[7]

When we examine a common product like a T-shirt and look for its many connections, we discover that it is wrapped around the world; it has touched many lives, some very negatively, and may have poisoned people, animals, and the natural resources upon which we all depend. The web of connections is far too complicated for us to gain more than a cursory understanding of a shirt's impact, but having even a glimpse allows us to open the door to different choices.

For example, an organic cotton T-shirt produced closer to home, without sweatshop labor, might have more positive consequences, as could a T-shirt purchased at a secondhand shop. A respectful letter to the CEO of a company that produces T-shirts

---

7. Much of the information on this "true cost" analysis of the cotton T-shirt comes from *Stuff: The Secret Lives of Everyday Things*, by John C. Ryan and Alan Thein Durning (Seattle, WA: Northwest Environmental Watch, 1997).

can influence that company's policies, especially if others write letters, too. And potentially, there is a fabric yet to be discovered that will not be destructive or energy intensive to produce, and will also biodegrade easily and nourish the earth when it's worn out. In addition to making considered consumer choices now, we can support those inventors and companies working to realize a better vision.

The act of making these outer connections requires an inner commitment. Being willing to inquire into the connections between our choices and their effects is one of the most important ingredients in doing the most good and the least harm. If we don't make the effort to do this, we will be hard-pressed to see connections because they are hidden and circuitous. And frankly, awareness of connections can sometimes interfere with our ease and pleasure—though not, I believe, with our joy.

As we become aware of connections, our integrity calls upon us to act accordingly, yet this can be challenging. I certainly don't always succeed at this task. It sometimes requires more effort than I'm willing to make to convince my son's sports teams to buy more expensive organic cotton T-shirts instead of conventional ones. My MOGO ethic often gets skewed toward what's most good for my family in the short term, rather than what's really best for us and everyone else in the long term.

And of course, I'm only using T-shirts as an example. Every choice and every issue of our time deserves my effort at making connections, and I know that it is often easier to close my eyes and cover my ears than to seek out information that would affect my emotional ease in being impulsive or satisfying my desires. Yet, despite the occasional interference with ease and pleasure, making connections is clearly worth it.

At the risk of repeating myself, a life lived succumbing to our impulses and surface desires is rarely satisfying, peaceful, or healthy, whereas the effort it takes to persevere toward higher goals is usually deeply satisfying. When we do choose to make connections, we actually save ourselves and so many others from persistent troubles. Plus, as soon as we imagine the creation of clothing (or any product) that benefits everyone, we may be filled with enthusiasm, hope, and excitement for ourselves and the future, tipping the balance toward joy over feelings of self-deprivation.

●●●

I read an interview with Gregg Krech, author of *Naikan: Gratitude, Grace, and the Japanese Art of Self-Reflection*, in *The Sun* magazine.[8] Deeply moved by the interview, I ordered the book and found it to be one of the most profound and important books I had ever read. The essence of *Naikan*, a Japanese word that means "looking inside," is a reflection on three simple questions:

- What have I received from _____?
- What have I given to _____?
- What troubles or difficulties have I caused _____?

Such questions don't seem so special, but try filling in the blank with some people—perhaps your family members, your teachers, your friends, or the people who produce your food, your clothes, and the products you use. Really ask and answer these questions. You are likely to discover that you have received more than you ever realized. Possibly, you will discover that you've given less than you've received, and you may even realize that you have caused others trouble that never occurred to you before.

In our family, we each say something for which we're grateful before we eat our dinner. Some nights, too many really, we fail to deeply reflect upon our gratitude. Perhaps we've had a disagreement that colors our gratitude, or a "bad" day. Yet, each evening we sit together with abundant food in a warm home in a beautiful part of the world, with our basic needs all met, and sometimes all we can muster is surface gratitude. When I step back to examine this, I'm astounded at how much easier it is to complain and feel like life isn't just the way I want it, instead of reveling in gratitude for all that I've been given.

---

8. Angela Winter, "Many Thanks: Gregg Krech on the Revolutionary Practice of Gratitude," *The Sun* (December 2004), 4.

As soon as I self-reflect on this pattern of disappointment, irritation, and frustration, I am able to pause and look through a different lens, one that illuminates the gifts, the opportunities, the possibilities for being different. In those moments, the call to give back sounds like a foghorn, deep and resonant, beckoning me out of my own myopia to live my life in service rather than expecting life to serve me.

The moment we become aware of the depth of our gratitude, we are lifted out of a sense of deprivation or victimization, and are humbled by the reality that so many others make our life possible. It is then that we may quicken our pace to give of ourselves and help others.

For twelve years our neighbor has plowed our driveway after a snowstorm. When he first stopped by, shortly after we'd moved into our house, we agreed upon a price for plowing. A couple of years later, when I received the bill after the first snowfall, the price had gone up a few dollars. The following season it went up several more dollars. I found myself irritated that the price had gone up two years in a row without my neighbor talking to me first, and so when he came by to plow one day, I asked him if it was going to keep going up at that rate each year. He was clearly put off by my question and invited me to find someone else to do the work if I thought I could get a cheaper price on plowing. I hastened to assure him I was happy to continue with his services, and that was the end of that.

Then I read the book *Naikan*, and it hit me like the proverbial ton of bricks: my neighbor had been getting up at 4:30 in the morning to plow after storms, and had plowed not once but sometimes several times during a storm to ensure that we could get in and out of our driveway (never charging more than half price for a second plowing and often nothing at all). While we were snug in bed, he was making it possible for us to come and go as we wished, no matter what the weather. The price for plowing had gone up about 7 percent since we moved in, and in that time the cost of fuel had gone up almost 20 percent. What had I been thinking? The truth was I hadn't been thinking and certainly not reflecting. I'd been wallowing in entitlement instead of recognizing what an enormous service my neighbor had been providing. I'd been feeling annoyed about a rise in price without my neighbor first talking to me about the increase, instead of realizing that my neighbor's expenses had been rising each year.

As soon as I saw how self-centered I'd been, I wrote my neighbor a thank you note and voluntarily increased the price I'd been paying him (fuel costs had continued to climb). Now that my eyes had been opened, I wanted to express my gratitude to my neighbor.

What does this have to do with MOGO living? If I self-reflect honestly, and take stock of what I've received and what I've given, I'm far less likely to treat others poorly, to see them as impediments to my happiness, or to see satisfying my every desire as a positive goal. Self-reflection humbles me, inspires me to give back more fully, and makes me pause before causing harm to others, be they other people, other species, or the environment. If I ask myself the third *Naikan* question: "What trouble or difficulties have I caused _____?" I'm more likely to consider living with greater respect, awareness, and kindness. I'm less likely to be blind to the effects of my actions and choices.

Honest self-reflection upon what we receive also creates an opportunity to gaze with wider eyes upon the realities of our choices and their effects. It further enables us to make connections. For example, imagine a man reflecting upon a breakfast of coffee, bacon, and eggs. He pauses to think about those who made his meal possible, and because he has sought to make connections, he realizes that some have become ill from exposure to pesticides on coffee plantations, and some rainforests were razed for monoculture coffee farms, and many birds disappeared when the rainforests were cut down. Then he thinks about the pigs and chickens who suffered enormously in factory farms, in transport to slaughterhouses, and during slaughter for the bacon and eggs in front of him. (Read more about factory farming in chapter 4, **Food**.)

The third *Naikan* question is like a whisper as he sits down to eat, begging him to consider the pain his choices have caused these others. He may find that he doesn't actually want to be part of such suffering and destruction. He may realize that he's not at all grateful that his choices contributed to harm. It is also possible he will quickly want to shut the door on this sort of unsettling thinking, but perhaps he will find himself ready to make different breakfast choices so that he can be truly grateful for what he receives instead of being burdened by the knowledge that his choices cause preventable suffering.

Are you thinking that self-reflection doesn't sound so joyful any more, that if being aware means feeling guilt, it's a lousy tradeoff? It takes effort to inquire and introspect, and honest self-reflection carries with it the potential for internal conflict. Some of our desires will inevitably compete with our values. There may be times when we do not want to do what we believe is right.

While such inner conflict may not sound appealing, I believe that avoiding reflection does not really serve us as well as we might think it does. There may be a superficial veneer of inner peace that comes with ignorance, but we can never be entirely immune from the harm and destruction that we participate in causing. Committing to self-reflection allows us to make both connections and choices that create real inner and outer peace, and to experience gratitude that is unhindered by shame or guilt.

In his book *Collapse: How Societies Choose to Fail or Succeed*, anthropologist, geographer, and historian Jared Diamond discusses a number of ancient and modern societies from all over the globe, revealing the common reasons why some collapsed and others succeeded. Consistently, the key to success has been farsightedness. Those societies that don't think ahead—those that deforest their land, erode their soil, drain their aquifers, and live in denial about the consequences of their choices—collapse; those that protect their resources and find peaceful means of interacting with other cultures usually survive for the long term.

For example, inhabitants of Easter Island, famous for its sculpted stone faces, exploited the island's resources and completely deforested it, resulting in societal collapse. The Pacific island nation Polynesian Tonga, on the other hand, has survived for thirty-two hundred years, extracting its resources no faster than they can be renewed. While none of the societies that Diamond examines is a model of perfect peacefulness by any means, successful cultures predictably follow an approach that works: thoughtful, considered, wise, nuanced, far-seeing, many-sided choice-making. They are societies in which people make connections, self-reflect, and choose wisely.

A final note about gratitude: in their brilliant and visionary book *Break Through: From the Death of Environmentalism to the Politics of Possibility*, authors Ted Nordhaus and Michael Shellenberger make the case that positive change doesn't usually emerge from scare tactics or guilt trips. It's possible that while you have been reading this chapter, you may have felt guilty about some of the pleasures that your good fortune allows which unwittingly cause suffering and destruction (such as the breakfast I described). This book makes the case that many of our ordinary choices cause preventable harm, and we can make new choices that do more good. This will then improve our own lives, bring us greater inner peace, and contribute to a better world. Nordhaus and Shellenberger invite us to view such choices in this way: "Those of us who are fortunate enough to have met our basic material and post-material needs should feel neither guilt nor shame at our wealth, freedom, and privilege, but rather *gratitude*. Whereas guilt drives us to deny our wealth, gratitude inspires us to share it."[9] The key is to make connections and self-reflect in such a way that we share our very best choices, systems, and structures so that all may thrive.

Practical Tips on Making Connections and Self-reflecting

- When you read or listen to the news, practice drawing connections between the issues of the day, and people's individual and societal choices.
- Seek out the answers to the questions that arise in your mind. Consider yourself an investigator who must find the clues to understand the causes of the problems around you.

---

9. Michael Shellenberger and Ted Nordaus, *Break Through: From the Death of Environmentalism to the Politics of Possibility* (Boston: Houghton Mifflin, 2007), 250.

- Choose a problem of our time and write down all the influencing factors you can think of. See how many connections you can make. Consider what would need to happen to solve the problem. Write down as many ideas as you can think of for solving the problem.
- Actively seek out many different sources of information for any problem or issue that concerns you. Do not to allow yourself to know only one side of an issue or to rely on only one news-and-information source, no matter how much you may have come to trust it.
- Practice the *Naikan* reflection described in this chapter by asking and answering the *Naikan* questions: What have I received from _____? What have I given to _____? What troubles or difficulties have I caused _____? (You might try this the first time right before bed, asking the questions about your day.)
- Make it a habit to thank others for specific services they provide. Imagine having twenty "thank yous" to give away each day, and then do so.

Key 4—Model Your Message and Work for Change

A mother brought her son to Mahatma Gandhi, begging Gandhi to persuade him to stop eating sugar as his doctor had recommended for his health. But instead of talking to the boy, Gandhi told the woman to come back in a couple of weeks. When she brought her son to Gandhi a few weeks later, Gandhi persuaded the boy to give up sugar. The mother was grateful, of course, but perplexed. Why, she asked Gandhi, had he made them wait? Gandhi replied that before he could tell anyone else to give up sugar, he had to give it up himself.

To create a peaceful world, we must each make our lives mirrors of the world we want. As nineteenth-century social reformer and minister William Ellery Channing stated, "May your life preach more loudly than your lips." Gandhi also responded to a reporter asking him what his message was by jotting down on a piece of paper, "My life is my message." There is much to do on the path to

MOGO living, but the foundation is laid when you make your life the message you want it to be.

A couple of years ago I attended a conference full of people who want to put an end to animal exploitation and abuse. Virtually all of us were angry about the institutionalized cruelty perpetrated on animals in our world, but a very small minority was especially vociferous in their attacks on people who participate in such cruelty. One went so far as to shout out, "I'm tired of people saying that factory farmers aren't bad people, they're just doing bad things. To those people I say, f— you! Factory farmers are bad people! Vivisectors are bad people!" My hand flew up in the air to respond. "With all due respect," I began, "then we are all 'bad' people. How many of us are wearing clothes produced in sweatshops or have eaten chocolate this weekend produced through slave labor? I married a vivisector, and he is now a veterinarian," I continued, before being interrupted by a woman who shouted out, "He was a bad person, and now he's a good person." Again, I asked if her shirt was produced in a sweatshop and if so, does that make her a bad person, and she loudly retorted, "That's not my issue."

I've been thinking about this exchange ever since. There are so many aspects that call for a response. First, there is the categorization and judgment of people as good or bad based on some of their behaviors, rather than assessing the behaviors themselves and assuming that people have the capacity to choose kindness if they are aware and empowered to do so. Then there is the belief that our particular "issues" are the only ones that are important, and we need not learn about other forms of suffering and exploitation happening in the world. Such limited thinking prevents us from listening, stretching, making connections, and ultimately creating a humane world for everyone. Lastly, name-calling doesn't achieve much more than defensiveness among the recipients of our anger. It doesn't create a more peaceful world. As Vaclav Havel wrote, "There is only one way to strive for decency, reason, responsibility, sincerity, civility, and tolerance, and that is decently, reasonably, responsibly, sincerely, civilly, and tolerantly."[10]

---

10. Vaclav Havel, *Summer Meditations* (New York: Vintage, 1993), 8.

There is a place for our anger. Anger is an appropriate emotional response to injustice, cruelty, or harm, and it can spark our commitment to create change. In the privacy of my home, and with my close friends and colleagues, I share my fury and pain over the destruction of this planet, the abuse we hurl upon the disenfranchised people around the globe, the horror we inflict upon animals, and the ways in which our culture hides the suffering in which we take part. I am not without judgment of those people who treat others, whether human or nonhuman, cruelly. It's nearly impossible for me not to judge the slave owner who forces a child to tie knots in rugs twelve hours a day, or the person who mercilessly beats a dog or pig. And I've certainly judged those CEOs of corporations who knowingly despoil this planet and exploit others. But I know that when I judge a person (as opposed to a behavior), I close the door on my ability to influence that person and create positive change, so I vent only with those closest to me and I try to understand how I might use my anger to propel me toward efforts that do good.

If our hearts are open to seeing suffering, they can easily break under the weight of so much pain in our world. Our anger may threaten to consume us and turn us into people who hate, even though it was our love that broke our hearts open to begin with. Yet the expression of hate achieves nothing positive: neither inner peace for ourselves nor a more peaceful world. As was written in the Buddhist *Dhammapada*, "Hatred can never put an end to hatred; love alone can."[11]

How we handle our despair and anger could be a book itself, but perhaps Joan Baez gave the best advice when she said, "Action is the antidote to despair." The key is to make certain that our actions truly model what we hope to achieve and what we really want. If we model antagonism and rage, we may set the stage for ineffective and sometimes counterproductive outcomes.

Modeling our message—"walking the talk"—may be the most challenging task before each of us. It is, in my mind, a spiritual

---

11. Eknath Easwaran, *God Makes the Rivers to Flow: Selections from the Sacred Literature of the World* (Tomales, CA: Nilgiri Press, 1992), 43.

discipline that is as demanding and difficult as any practice could ever be. It begins with being kind, respectful, and honest in our interactions, but it doesn't end there. Modeling your message also entails making choices about products, clothing, transportation, recreation, food, volunteerism, and work that reflect your values and are peaceful, humane, restorative, and sustainable. How difficult this can be to actually do! But what a rich and rewarding practice it is to model your message. I'm not suggesting that you can or will always succeed in every moment, but you can consistently try. (There is more about how to do this in part II, "Choosing Outward.")

I practice the martial art of Aikido. It is unlike most other martial arts because we do not learn how to attack or harm others. Instead, we practice diffusing violent or aggressive acts using the energy from attackers to stop them from harming us, without harming them in return. We transform violence into safety by staying centered, blending, and removing ourselves from harm's way. Rather than block an attack and follow with a counterattack, an Aikidoist often circles out of the way, prevents the attacker from causing harm, and either pins or throws the attacker in such a way as to stop the aggression by using the attacker's own energy—again without harm. By blending my movement with my attackers', I not only protect myself, I also face the same direction as they. Suddenly, I see the world from their perspective.

How does Aikido relate to MOGO living? So often we perceive others as opponents. In fact, our culture consistently perpetuates either/or scenarios. In the United States there is a two-party political system, as if there are only two perspectives on government policies. States are either called red or blue. The media present issues in either/or terms as well (i.e., either we save the Northern Spotted Owl or loggers lose their jobs). But what if we were to approach others in a different way? What if we were to blend, hear others out, and see the world from their perspective? Chances are we would realize that we have more in common than we thought, and we would find more effective ways to respond to conflicts. We would uncover wiser choices to solve seemingly intractable problems.

In Aikido there are literally thousands of combinations of techniques that one can use when attacked. Those thousands of choices allow the Aikidoist to choose based on the situation; not from a fixed and immutable position, but from the actual experience of conflict and looking from the other's perspective.

One morning I was listening to *Morning Edition* on National Public Radio. The reporter was recounting a situation in which a teacher was fired for failing a couple of students on their lab reports because they had slept through class. Although the students produced good reports, the teacher had explained at the beginning of the semester that student participation was part of their grade. The parents of the students were upset that the teacher had failed their children and went to the school board, which ruled in the parents' favor. The teacher was fired.

When I heard this story, I was dismayed yet again by my society's practice of choosing sides, and creating winners and losers. While I don't know the details of this situation beyond what was reported on the radio, I do know that there are many more options than failing students for sleeping during class, or firing a teacher for failing those students. There are so many questions to ask: Why were the students sleeping during class? Why were they so tired? Were they bored? How late were they staying up doing homework? How early must they rise for school? Are the subjects we're teaching teenagers the most important ones for their lives and for our society? Are grades the best way to ensure attentiveness, involvement, and learning? What could the teacher, students, parents, and administrators have done differently? What alternatives are there to failing the students? To firing the teacher? These questions came to mind immediately upon hearing the report, but the reporter did not address any of them. Instead the report presented a win/lose conflict.

I recount this story because I believe that when we fall into the trap of choosing sides instead of striving for positive solutions to conflicts and problems, we model something different from peace; we model antagonistic thinking. The book *The Third Side*, by William Ury, explores a problem-solving approach to conflict in which we always seek an alternative to the two sides presented to us. The very concept of a third side is a powerful perspective to bring to every situation in which conflict arises because it calls upon us to find a way out of two-sided thinking. Certainly there can be more than three sides, too. By seeking the third side, or the fourth and fifth, we might find ourselves discovering brilliant answers to both small and large problems. If more of us modeled this sort of complex and nuanced thinking, I believe that the world around us would begin to change in positive ways.

For example, the media might find that either/or presentations stopped attracting as many listeners and viewers, and they might focus on reporting about solutions to problems and conflicts. Politicians might discover that "us versus them" campaigns are no longer successful at gaining votes, whereas solution-oriented plans for the future win elections. When the day comes that we aren't drawn to or satisfied with messages that pit us against one another (these people against those people; people versus the environment; the environment versus individual animals; people versus animals), we will discover that we have always had the tools to make choices that can largely benefit everyone. There will certainly always be conflicts, and short-term desires will still clash with long-term needs, but there will be better answers that serve all interests, as long as we are willing to seek them out, see the world from others' perspectives, and strive for solutions in which everyone's needs are met.

Given the complexities of our society and the ways in which our lives—no matter how scattered across the globe—are entwined, modeling MOGO in all our behaviors and relationships, especially those relationships that are woven in a complicated web (such as our relationship with oil, building materials, or something as simple as a cup of coffee), is a hugely challenging endeavor.

Recently my friend and colleague Dani Dennenberg sent out a group email asking about where she might find a blender produced sustainably and equitably—without sweatshop labor, without packaging that is destructive, or transportation that is unsustainable. She received several replies: one suggesting that she look for a used blender, another advocating a hand-cranked blender, another asking whether she really needed a blender at all. The reality is that it wasn't easy for Dani to find what she wanted because we haven't yet created a world in which the norm for companies is to produce environmentally friendly, equitably produced products that do not rely upon unsustainable energy sources, and unecological production and disposal.

Dani has another option as well. In addition to trying to model her message personally, she can also work to influence company policies. She can recognize that it is not always possible to be a perfect consumer whose purchases have no ill effects, but it is possible to create a vision of equity and sustainability, exercise her voice by promoting and working for such a vision, and engage herself politically—all to promote substantive changes. Dani's individual choice of a blender is only one ingredient in modeling her message. Her effort in change-making is equally important.

As Eban Goodstein, an economics professor at Lewis and Clark College, has written:

> Government—our collective voice—has consistently made the morally wrong choices, subsidizing big fossil fuel producers and failing to support clean energy technologies. Not as individual consumers but as a political society, we have failed to demand increased fuel efficiency in our vehicles, and as a result we see our oil dollars fund terrorism in the Middle East, our young people suffer from an asthma crisis in our cities, and our planet's climate grow increasingly unstable.
>
> If, instead of focusing on the need for change . . . we talk about our neighbor's lifestyle choices, most of us can rightly be charged with failing—miserably—to practice what we preach. More importantly, blaming instead of engaging our neighbors will get us nowhere. Global warming will not be solved by lifestyle changes or any shift to simple living, desirable as those changes might be. We need to pledge our lives, our creative energies, and our broad-ranging collective talents to creating a political movement powerful enough, in a few short years, to launch

the new clean energy markets and global forest preservation efforts that will mark the beginning of the end of the fossil fuel era."[12]

I hope you will not read the above as an excuse not to make personal choices that reflect your values and model your message, because this is not an either/or scenario. Our individual choices are essential to the process of change. If we ourselves fail to model our message, we not only threaten our own inner peace and diminish our integrity, we also have less influence on others because we don't walk our proverbial talk. But Goodstein's central point is crucial. We must engage in change-making at the macro level. That is why this key to MOGO living is to both model your message *and* work for change. They are not two separate keys but rather two components of the same idea.

That Dani raised the question about appliances, and that several people responded with suggestions, while not a solution by itself, is a key to the solution. We can each do our best to model our message through our daily MOGO choices, and we can also support change by asking questions that inspire better answers, and by speaking out and participating in democracy, volunteerism, and activism.

Somewhere an inventor is working and innovating to discover a better, more environmentally friendly blender (or form of transportation, or source of fuel). If you are one of the people searching for innovations (or innovating yourself), you're speeding up the process of change and helping create a peaceful, sustainable planet. Simultaneously, there are politicians emerging and supporters to help them gain office, as well as profit-minded businesspeople, who want to make the creation of sustainable systems and products the norm. It will be a combination of sane, doable, joyful, personal choice-making that best models your message, and effort, and action to make those messages take hold in society that create both inner and outer peace.

---

12. Eban Goodstein, "What the World Needs Now is … Politics," *WorldWatch Magazine* (January/February 2006).

In their book, *Cradle to Cradle*, William McDonough and Michael Braungart offer a visionary challenge to those who seek to safeguard this planet and all its inhabitants. Rather than simply protesting what is wrong, painting a gloom-and-doom picture, or working on single-issue fixes to specific problems, entrepreneurs like McDonough and Braungart are envisioning and creating systems and products in which nothing is wasted, and nothing becomes trash or a pollutant. Their entire philosophy is based upon the development of products that are regenerative and nourishing. Asking the question, "How can we care for all children of all species for all time?" they create products, buildings, and systems that are not simply less destructive but are actually regenerative. Even their book is an innovation, made not from trees but from a polymer whose ink can be removed, without toxic solvents, so the pages can be reused and turned into a new book. Through their respective fields in architecture and chemistry, they are brilliant at both modeling their message *and* creating systemic change by developing "cradle to cradle"—rather than "cradle to grave"—products. McDonough and Braungart are working with the Ford Motor Company, the Gap, universities, some major cities, and others to create a completely different paradigm for positive change. They design home construction that doesn't deplete resources or include toxins, and which actually produces oxygen and nutrients. They're helping Ford to conceptualize cars that no longer pollute with nitrous oxide while generating the valuable nutrient, nitrogen.

More and more visionaries and leaders are imagining, modeling, and creating a new paradigm: one that doesn't just fight individual battles unconnected to the whole or simply demand endless restraint from citizens. This new paradigm envisions increased job opportunities through the creation of systems that will solve or diminish interconnected problems of global climate change, poverty, disease, exploitation of humans and animals, loss of biodiversity, and more.

Given this good news we might ask why we continue to have so many problems. Why, for example, do we still have automobile companies (such as Ford) producing gas-guzzling vehicles when the technology exists to do better, and when the commitment exists among many to create transportation that is more than just better—that is actually healthy? Why do we still measure our economic well-being by the amount of spending that takes place, even if that spending includes cleaning up oil spills or treating cancer patients? Why haven't we developed viable alternatives to fossil fuels when we know that eventually we must? Why haven't we sought out the third side more often? Why haven't more politicians committed to long-term thinking, or more to the point, why haven't we elected those politicians who do? Why haven't we, as individuals and as a culture, chosen to live according to our deepest values and to best model our message?

I believe the answer to these questions is two-fold. First, we do not always have good systems in place that facilitate and promote wise choices. For example, we allow special interests and corporations to fund politicians, thereby influencing policies for the short-term gain of a few. Corporations are not held accountable for the harm they cause; rather, they are held accountable for the profits they provide shareholders. These are just two examples illustrating why we must work for changes in systems in addition to modeling our personal message. Secondly, as both individuals and within societies, we too often succumb to our propensity toward denial, myopia, and greed—natural enough responses for humans but not inevitable responses, and certainly not representative of our range of choices.

Denial is a complicated psychological state that can lead to terrible decision-making, and consequent suffering and destruction. However, denial is also very useful when faced with situations that cause significant fear, anxiety, and sorrow. I believe that our denial keeps us sane in a world full of suffering, allowing us to forget so that we can satisfy our longing for joy, avoid the unbearable, and gratify our desires in the face of realities we may find overwhelming. It is important, however, not to allow denial, myopia, and the incessant fulfillment of our immediate desires to eclipse our deeper wish to live in a peaceful, humane, and sustainable society on a healthy planet. That is why the effort to model our message and work for change is so crucial.

Practical Suggestions to Better Model Your Message and Work for Change

- Make the phrase "My life is my message" a mantra. Repeat it often so that you have more awareness of your actions and choices, and are more likely to model the message you want.
- Count to ten before you react to anything that makes you angry. Take a deep breath. Repeat the mantra. Choose to act peacefully and wisely.
- Whenever you are exposed to either/or thinking, whether in the media, with family or friends, or in yourself, commit to discovering other perspectives. Pause to explore solutions.
- Always search for alternatives to violence, whether violent words, violent acts, or violent attitudes. Uncover a third way. If necessary, uncover a fourth or fifth.
- Practice blending. When facing a conflict or challenge, whether with others or within yourself, listen carefully and pay attention to the other point(s) of view before reacting or responding.
- Reflect upon and celebrate the times you have successfully modeled your message so that you may call upon your own wisdom, integrity, and creativity the next time you are faced with a challenge or conflict.
- You will find many suggestions for ways to work for change in chapter 6, **Activism, Volunteerism, and Democracy**. Choose those that most engage and enthuse you.
- Make sure to complete the **MOGO Questionnaire and Action Plan** in part III, and follow through with your commitments and goals.

Key 5—Find and Create Community

Striving to lead a MOGO life generally takes us at least somewhat out of the mainstream. Once we begin to question the products we use, the food we eat, the clothing we wear, the transportation we rely upon, the work we do, and the ways in which we engage in change (more about these in part II, "Choosing Outward"), we are called upon to make choices that are different from most that are advertised and actively promoted to us.

When we write our epitaph and commit to living our values; when we find that pursuing joy has nothing to do with the things we buy but everything to do with how we give to others; when we make connections and take the time to self-reflect; and when we commit to modeling our message and working for change, we discover that we're on a different path from the one that has been sold to us by a culture that compels us to fill up our time and fulfill our inner longings with excesses of food and pleasure-seeking, television and other entertainments, and endless products.

Once we realize that we have stepped off the wide boulevard of flashy lights vying for our attention and turned toward a more conscious MOGO path, we need to find community. Community is a broad concept, but a MOGO community can start very small— with just a friend, family member, or a colleague. Ideally, it will grow to be a vital, sustaining community of many people working together. It is rarely as healthy, satisfying, or effective to walk the MOGO path alone as it is to find others to go on the journey with us. There are millions of people on the MOGO path, seeking better answers to the problems we face, searching for meaningful work and opportunities to serve, and eschewing materialism; you will find them and draw them to yourself not only because it's MOGO for you to do so but because, in order to change systems that are destructive into ones that are restorative, we need groups of dedicated, wise, and visionary people.

I have a fifteen-year-old son, and there are nights when I go to bed feeling so much frustration about how our culture works against me as a parent, making family life unnecessarily conflictual. For example, I don't want my son eating junk food and drinking soda. I don't want him listening to misogynistic and violent lyrics on his iPod. But I don't want to police his every action either; I want him to make healthy, humane choices. I give him the tools and information to do so, but I'm competing with opposing societal and peer messages. I feel overpowered at times. Without other parents who share my values, and with whom I can create healthier standards and work for change, my task would be even greater. I rely upon this community of parents because it makes raising a humane child much easier.

Active involvement in communities helps create change on the micro level that can impact the macro level. For example, groups of frustrated parents and teachers have created innovative and successful schools that now serve as models for other communities. Some communities have created alternative economies in which community "dollars" promote local trade in goods and services. Others have supported local agriculture, organic farms, and farmers' markets.

There are thousands of examples of people working together in communities to develop better systems, whether in schooling, farming, economics, transportation, elder care, energy use, or waste management. Many of these people once felt isolated and alone in their beliefs and values, but they eventually found and/or created support for the journey they had begun.

It is possible that your current community of family and friends may not choose to support you in making changes in your life in the way you would like. Let's say that you read this book and decide that you want to eat differently. Will you have the support to make different choices? Perhaps you will want to do different things than you have in the past with your spare time. Will you have friends to join you? You may be the first person you know personally who cares about the issues you care about. You may be the first you know reading this book, or the first to make the choices you're making outside of the mainstream. It is even possible you've pushed people away in your effort to cultivate them as allies. I certainly did. When I first learned about factory farming, for example, I alienated a number of people by commenting (negatively) on their food choices. Instead of creating a supportive community, I isolated myself further. Not MOGO. Think of yourself as being not only on the cutting edge but on the leading edge; you are leading others toward healthy community.

So how can you find and cultivate community? Remember Melissa, Khalif, and Kim from **Key 1—Live Your Epitaph**? Each of them has a strong sense of community, even though community means different things to them. Melissa has a partner who lives in a different state. He shares her values and they fully support each other's efforts to make MOGO choices, even though they are separated by quite a distance. Melissa's mother and brother are also active members of her community, and they all support each other's efforts, too. But her mother lives in Philadelphia and her brother in Paris, France. In other words, Melissa's community is spread out but still very much a part of her support system. Her daily life in Boston includes active involvement in a variety of communities—some created around friendships, others around her teaching, others around her volunteer efforts—and consists of people she meets through daily life, such as Barbara, the refugee from Liberia whom she befriended after an exchange on the subway.

Kim also has friends, family, and a partner as well as colleagues who support her, and she has taken the concept of community another step. She has been actively engaged with a city garden that does more than grow vegetables. It is a meeting place for learning and exchanging ideas about MOGO living. She has also created an organization to bring together members of the community who work on a range of social change efforts. Through her organization, they can better understand the interconnections between their missions and spread a more holistic vision that will make each one of their individual goals more likely to succeed.

As for Khalif, his rural community in Maine has created an alternative economy that exists side by side with the global economy. Not only has Khalif been part of creating a vital extended family of friends who work and play together, but the sharing of time, skills, services, and products means that this community replaces the constant exchange of money with neighbor-to-neighbor bartering and sharing. Someone helps him build his house, and he helps another member of the community construct a timber frame hostel; they, in turn, help someone clear land for a vegetable garden, which then provides food for many. Melissa, Kim, and Khalif create community in different ways, but what they all have, and what all of us need, is support for and practice in engaging in MOGO living.

For most of human history we have lived within small communities. Sometimes these communities have constrained individuals in oppressive ways; shunning, ostracism, excommunication, disowning—these are the shadow side of community. Sometimes communities become insular, fighting other communities that are different. But the positive aspects of a healthy community include responsibility and compassion for its members.

Small community living is in decline, however, as more people move to large cities. Yet as Kim and Melissa demonstrate, positive community-building is not only possible in cities but also brings together diverse populations of people. Cities may often be crowded, polluted, and sometimes dangerous, and city living can often interfere with trust and connection, yet healthy communities can and do flourish in urban environments. Since cities are far more energy efficient per capita, often don't require individuals to own cars, and offer many economic opportunities, urban renewal presents the prospect of community-building and change-making.

Urban gardens, like the one Kim has been involved in, bring together neighbors in addition to providing local, fresh, and affordable produce. In Portland, Maine, a nonprofit organization called Cultivating Community brings gardens to neighborhoods and schools throughout the city, thereby cultivating both community and food. And more and more CSA (Community-Supported Agriculture) sites are available in cities, too. When I lived in Philadelphia I joined a CSA through my local food co-op. In April, I paid several hundred dollars to the farmer offering the CSA, and once a week throughout the growing season, I went to the co-op after work to pick up a box stuffed with seasonal vegetables and fruits from the farm. The affordable food was organic and produced nearby, and was therefore more nutritious and more environmentally friendly than pesticide-sprayed food that had traveled a couple thousand miles. But just as wonderful as the food was the community that formed around the CSA. I met more of my neighbors, connected with the person who was growing much of my food, and felt more embedded in my community, which was deeply satisfying and rewarding.

In chapter 6, **Activism, Volunteerism, and Democracy**, you'll read about Mohammad Yunus, who has helped millions of people in Bangladesh escape poverty through his Grameen Bank and microcredit movement. In the context of this chapter, however, Yunus's approach works because of a key factor: community. Grameen requires that a community of borrowers be responsible for ensuring that each individual's business project is viable and successful. It is the community of individuals that joins together to make certain that each individual succeeds.

We may start on the MOGO path alone, but we won't stay on it alone. We will inevitably either find or actively create a community with which to work, share, interact, and make a difference. But even this larger MOGO community isn't an end point. Ultimately the world is our community, and we must learn to live in harmony with everyone and the entire biosphere. We may need support for our journey in the form of individuals, but ultimately we must embrace the concept of community in an expansive way in order to create lasting peace for all.

If we can practice living well within smaller communities, we have the tools with which to practice living well on the planet. Although it is impossible to be aware of all our myriad interactions within the planetary community, we can still recognize that the earth needs us to be responsible inhabitants. Even though we may not be wired to be consciously cognizant of many connections without significant effort, we can still commit ourselves to being better members of both our local and global communities, and do the work it takes to succeed at this task.

Khalif is deeply embedded in his local community, drawing his energy from and putting his energy toward the place he has chosen as home by living simply, trading, sharing, and purchasing locally. He does this in large part to protect the global community. Melissa also became aware of how her choices were affecting the global community, but she chooses to actively engage with that global community, consciously using fair trade products and clothes produced by people working in collectives around the world whose lives she hopes to influence positively.

Embracing community can, and I would argue *must*, be local, national, and global. Just as we prepare a dinner for a community family that is faced with hardship, illness, or the birth of a new child, we can give to others farther removed and perceive everyone as our extended neighbor.

Modern media has enabled us to be aware of our faraway "neighbors." When natural disasters strike, the outpouring from the world to the victims is usually quite profound. We are able to extend our sense of community beyond our towns, states, provinces, and nations to help those in need. But we need not wait for disasters to be good global neighbors. All it takes for generosity to flow is awareness. By actively pursuing awareness and knowledge, we can make choices that cause less harm and greater good to others in the global community of our shared earth. Once we think of everyone on this planet as deserving of the same care and kindness as our neighbors next door, we will have an enduring perspective that not only motivates our compassion but also inhibits our capacity to cause harm.

We humans are good at rankings and divisions. We divide ourselves into groups based on class, color, religion, age, tribe, education, sexual orientation, intelligence, wealth, and talent. But we do not have to make these divisions the basis of either our communities or our actions and ethics. I suspect that it is not in our nature to be so inclusive. As Joshua Greene, professor of psychology at Harvard University, says, "The idea that you can save the life of a stranger on the other side of the world ... is not the kind of situation our social brains are prepared for."[13]

Human histories, countless societies, and numerous studies of social psychology suggest that we are not inclined to welcome strangers, accept differences, or share with outsiders. But we *are* able to do so, and for every hate crime or genocide, there are examples of altruism—of humans reaching beyond borders, race, religion, and class to create a planetary community. Someday, I hope that we will all be patriots of our planet and not just of our respective nations. And I hope that we will be able to demon-

---

13. Quoted in Jeffrey Kluger, "What Makes Us Normal," *Time* (December 3, 2007): 58.

strate our altruism and kindness in everyday choices, not only during crises.

We can also extend our circle of community to include animals. As just one example of our failure to consider animals, consider what happened during Hurricane Katrina, which struck the Gulf States in the United States in 2005. Rescue workers told evacuees that they could not bring their animals with them. When a young boy's dog was wrenched out of his arms before the boy was permitted to board a rescue bus, something truly dreadful happened, and it wasn't just to the dog. That boy, who we can only assume had already gone to great lengths to save his dog, was taught a horrifying lesson about responsibility and community.

When I heard about this scene—played out on national television news—I could imagine the aftereffects. The boy may well have survived emotionally intact after losing his home and enduring extremes of horror many of us can barely fathom, but he might not fully recover from having his beloved dog, whom he had made such an effort to protect, pulled from his arms and left to die in the flooded city.

It was not only companion dogs and cats who were excluded from the worthy-of-rescue community during Katrina.[14] Millions of animals were left to drown, suffocate, or starve in the wake of the hurricane. These included chickens, pigs, cows, and turkeys confined in cages and warehouse-like factory farms; and monkeys, rabbits, (as well as less beloved "research" dogs and cats) in the laboratories at Louisiana State University and elsewhere.[15] This one example is representative of how we generally treat animals, whether during natural disasters or daily life. We fail to consider them as being members of our communities.

The division we've set up between ourselves and other species is perhaps the most difficult to break down. Even the most vocal

---

14. Even our language excludes animals from care and concern. My word processing program, for example, underlined the word "who" in this sentence because dogs and cats are not considered "whos" in our grammar but rather "thats."

15. Leana Stormont, "Help Was Never on the Way," *Satya* (November 2005): http://www.satyamag.com/nov05/stormont.html.

opponents of bigotry and prejudice have too often failed to recognize the arbitrariness of our oppression, exploitation, and cruelty toward other sentient beings. We humans have managed to exclude from our community of care all the other species with whom we share this planet, with the exception of those individual animals we choose to love as "pets" and those we have designated as endangered (and now, even protections for endangered species are threatened). In so doing, we have created horrific systems of cruelty and exploitation that annually cause suffering and death to tens of billions of animals capable of feeling pain and fear, just like us. If we stop short of including other animals in our circles of community, I believe that we ultimately fail at the challenge of living truly MOGO lives.

In order to embrace animals as members of our community, we again need to use the 3 Is. While most of us love and care for our dogs and cats, our culture and media do not encourage us to inquire about the effects of our choices on other animals. Since it is easier to remain ignorant of the effects of our individual and societal choices on other species, many of us don't make an effort to inquire. But as soon as we do, we learn not only that our world has deeply entrenched systems of cruelty and exploitation, but that there also are numerous groups, organizations, and even businesses seeking to end such cruelty and create humane systems, products, and societies. We then have the opportunity to introspect, determine how we would like to live in relation to other species, and practice integrity through both our daily choices (what we eat, wear, and buy) and our efforts at participating in positive change for animals.

The tools and values that allow us to live successfully within small communities—awareness, generosity, trust, caring—are the same tools and values that enable us to live with respect for the planetary community. Living humanely in relationship to distant communities that supply our food, minerals, energy sources, building materials, clothing, transportation, telecommunications, electronics, and other products is not easy, but it is necessary to try if we want to create a peaceful, sustainable world and live a MOGO life.

Practical Ways to Find Others to Go on the MOGO Journey with You

📝 Share this book with a friend or family member, or donate it to your local library, adding your name and email address in the space provided on the last page so others can contact you. In this way, you can create a community of people interested in MOGO living.

📝 Go to meetings or join organizations of people working on some of the issues addressed in this book.

📝 Post a note at your local library, food co-op, or other community-based center, inviting people interested in MOGO living to meet.

Practical Ways to Involve Yourself Within Local Communities

📝 Become more engaged and active in your community by:
- Running for local office or supporting someone who is
- Helping in a community garden
- Volunteering at a local food pantry
- Volunteering at your local animal shelter
- Joining a volunteer fire department or neighborhood watch
- Participating in neighborhood clean-ups
- Joining a local food co-op, community garden, or CSA. You can find a CSA near you by visiting thegreenguide.com.
- Frequenting your local library, reading the posted notices about events, and attending some of them
- Joining the PTA if you are a parent
- Starting or joining a MOGO school club if you are a student (visit HumaneEducation.org for more information)
- Becoming a member of a spiritual/religious community that reflects your beliefs and values
- Creating a MOGO living group at your elder facility

While some of the groups listed above provide opportunities for involvement and action, they may not always create a sense of real community. That may be something that you can bring to them, however, through your own joyful engagement.

🌿 Help neighbors and friends by:
- Cooking and shopping for them when needed
- Exchanging childcare or babysitting
- Shoveling snow, stacking wood, and clearing downed trees when necessary
- Walking dogs for those who are homebound due to illness or injury
- Sharing what you have that might be of use to neighbors[16]
- Passing along outgrown clothes and/or toys
- Hosting a clothing or other product exchange

🌿 Get your community's pollution report card. Visit: score card.org, type in your zip code, and immediately receive details about who is polluting in your county and region. With this information, you'll be able to follow up on the site's suggestions for actions.

Practical Ways to Pursue Living MOGO in Relation to the Planetary Community

🌿 Create or join community groups that work on global issues. For example, if you're inspired to help political prisoners, you can join local groups that write letters for Amnesty International (amnesty.org). Or maybe you want to put an end to child labor by becoming involved with neighbors and friends in various campaigns and efforts (stopchildlabor.org). There are organizations working to end genocide, factory farming, and pollution; protecting rainforests and whales; and challenging corruption in government and in the corporate world (see chapter 12, **Recommended Resources**, for information on organizations and websites). Whatever your passion, find a group of like-minded people,[17] and become involved in creating a better global community while building a local community for yourself.

---

16. Visit http://www.neighborrow.com.

17. Visit http://www.meetup.com to find a group near you that's focused on issues of mutual concern.

🖋 Become knowledgeable about the products you use and buy by asking:
- Where did this product come from?
- Who or what may have been harmed to produce this product (including other humans, animals, and the environment)?
- What product would do the most good and the least harm?

🖋 Become knowledgeable about the foods you eat by asking:
- Where did this food come from?
- Who or what may have been harmed to produce this food (including other humans, animals, and the environment)?
- What foods would do the most good and the least harm?

🖋 See the chapters **Products** and **Food** that cover these issues in detail, and part III, which provides resources for answering these questions.

Key 6—Take Responsibility

In the early 1960s, psychologist Stanley Milgram performed what have become infamous experiments on obedience to authority. Answering an ad that offered $4.50 for one hour's work, people participated in what were described as studies to examine the influence of punishment on learning.

Meeting a stern experimenter and an affable cosubject, each pair of participants picked a slip of paper to see who would be the "learner" and who would be the "teacher." The teacher was told to administer shocks to the learner, sequestered in another room, whenever he failed to answer a question correctly, and to increase the level of shock each time the learner answered incorrectly. The switches that administered the shock indicated the voltage (ranging from 15 to 450 volts in 15-volt increments) and included a rating from "slight shock" to "danger: severe shock." The last two switches were labeled "XXX." The teacher could hear the cries of the learner when he pressed switches that administered high voltages. As the voltage increased, the learner pleaded for the shocks to stop and referred to his heart condition. Many of the teachers became worried and upset by what they were doing, but once they were told that the experimenter assumed all responsibility, they continued to increase the shocks to the learner.

What the teachers did not know was that they themselves were the actual test subjects, that the victim of the electric shocks was simply an actor who was not, in fact, getting shocked, and that the slips of paper to determine who would be teacher and who would be learner were rigged. Unbeknownst to the teachers, the study was not examining the effects of punishment on learning but rather their own obedience to authority.

The results of the study were *truly* shocking. No teacher stopped before pressing the switch that indicated 300 volts of electricity, and a whopping 65 percent of the teachers were willing to obey the orders of the experimenter to deliver the maximum level of shock, thinking that they were harming and possibly even killing the learner who, by the maximum voltage, made no sound at all.

Dr. Milgram concluded that the essence of obedience consists in the fact that a person comes to view himself as the instrument for carrying out another person's wishes, and therefore no longer regards himself as responsible for his own actions. This conclusion may explain a host of atrocities, the most famous of which was the willingness of so many ordinary German people to carry out the Holocaust during World War II.

But our unwillingness to take responsibility for our actions goes even further. It is not only for the sake of others' wishes that we often fail to accept our responsibility; we also frequently refuse to acknowledge that we bear responsibility for others' suffering when we carry out our *own* wishes.

Each day we wake up and make myriad choices that affect others. We clothe ourselves with shirts, pants, and shoes that may have been sewn together by women working in factories fourteen-plus hours a day for a nonliving wage; we buy products manufactured in ways that destroy forests, pollute waterways, and poison the air; we wash our hair with shampoos that may have been squeezed into the eyes of conscious rabbits or force-fed to them in quantities that kill; and on and on. As Derrick Jensen has written in his book *The Culture of Make Believe*, "It is possible to kill a million people without personally shedding a drop of blood. It is possible to destroy a culture without being aware of its existence. It is possible to commit genocide or ecocide from the comfort of one's living room."

I too, am guilty of this renunciation of responsibility, too often failing to acknowledge and therefore change much of the destruction I leave in my wake. Why do we all (to greater and lesser degrees) choose not to take responsibility for the suffering our choices cause? We might say:

- My individual choices don't matter.
- Corporations are responsible, not I.
- It's the way of the world, and I can't stop it.
- These problems will get worked out over time.
- Sweatshop jobs may be bad, but they are better than no jobs, and I'm contributing to employment.
- Animals can't really feel and suffer the way we do, and they don't have souls, so I do not have to consider their pain.
- Environmental problems are probably overblown.
- Technology and inventions will solve our environmental problems anyway.
- I like certain foods and clothes, and I'm not willing to give them up.
- Boycotts don't work.
- I can't afford the products produced environmentally and humanely.
- I don't have time to learn about all these issues.
- I don't want to change.
- I'm too lazy.
- Someone else will fix things.

Even if we do not actually articulate these thoughts or feelings, many of them probably exist in some nonverbal form in our psyches, keeping us from learning and choosing more kindly and wisely. But if you're reading this book, presumably you *do* want to learn about and make MOGO choices. Maybe some of the issues I touched upon above (product choices, food choices, clothing choices) are ones that you consider in your life. Perhaps you are an advocate of human rights, environmental preservation, or animal protection, or are part of a movement that is challenging our materialistic society or the effects of media monopolies. Perhaps you try to make MOGO food choices but not clothing choices. Maybe you involve yourself with social justice issues but not environmental issues. Perhaps you simply want a better world.

Whatever your concerns and motivations, it would be surprising if you were able to make conscious, examined, and deliberate choices on every issue related to MOGO living because there are so many issues to know about, and the intricacies of our lives necessarily impact many others about whom we are largely, and understandably, unaware. Even when we do know about all these interconnected issues and care immensely, it's still not possible to cause no harm at all.

Yet each of us—you and I and everyone who is privileged enough to actually make consumer, political, career, recreation, and lifestyle choices—is still responsible for the effects of our choices, and we are responsible for creating a government that ensures protections to those without power, freedom, or speech. Maybe we cannot easily find a pair of athletic shoes that is not produced in a sweatshop, but that doesn't mean we can't exercise our voice, contact the companies that produce these shoes with our concerns or write to our legislators to urge that laws be passed to prevent the exploitation of foreign workers by multinationals. And while we cannot avoid causing animal suffering entirely, we can avoid causing animal cruelty in obvious ways where we do have choices.

We may not be able to single-handedly create a peaceful world, but we can still strive to live without causing avoidable violence and destruction as much as we are able. And although we cannot solve every problem, this doesn't mean we cannot become politically active and visionary in our thinking to advance meaningful, positive change.

Another social psychologist, Dr. Philip Zimbardo, conducted an experiment at Stanford University in 1971 in which participating male college students, who were carefully screened for mental health, were divided into two groups—prisoners and guards—in a makeshift jail created in the basement of Stanford's psychology building. The experiment was set to last two weeks, but Dr. Zimbardo had to call it off after six days, and only after an outside observer brought the horror of what had happened to his attention. He, as the "warden" in the experiment, had become so caught up in the experiment himself that he failed to intervene to stop the cruelty and suffering his mock jail had created. In fact, it had taken no more than forty-eight hours before some guards began acting in a sadistic manner, and some prisoners became powerless and physically ill victims, despite the fact that any participant could leave the experiment at any time. Dr. Zimbardo has written about the experiment and its aftermath in detail in his 2007 book, *The Lucifer Effect*, and one of the salient points that he makes is that there are three components to determining our behaviors: the person, the situation, and the system.

So far in this chapter, I've urged you as the reader to take responsibility for your choices, arguing that as an individual you have the ethical obligation to do so. Perhaps you found it shocking that so many participants in Dr. Milgram's experiments actually pressed the levers they believed might seriously injure or kill their compatriots who signed up for a simple experiment. What both Dr. Milgram's and Dr. Zimbardo's experiments and analyses reveal, however, is that although we as individuals do have the capacity to take responsibility for our actions and choices, they will be influenced significantly by the situations we are in and the systems that surround us.

Each of us is embedded within political, economic, social, religious, and family systems that constrain us and subtly influence our individual choices. We are also embedded within specific situations that affect our behaviors and decisions. The participants in Dr. Zimbardo's experiment were constrained by the prison system that was created for them, and then they were further influenced by the specific situation in which they were placed, as a prisoner or as a guard. The system and the situation were so powerful that everyone's individual thoughts, feelings, and behaviors were dramatically altered—even Dr. Zimbardo's.

Hannah Arendt, a political theorist, coined the phrase "the banality of evil" in discussing how ordinary people, believing that their actions are simply normal, participate in atrocities such as the Holocaust. Dr. Zimbardo has recently coined a new phrase: "the banality of heroism." If ordinary people can become perpetrators of evil, so, too, can ordinary people become heroes. But we need to create changes in systems and situations in order to make ordinary heroism ubiquitous.

Some of us live within extremely challenging and sometimes completely debilitating social, political, and economic systems and situations; others live within problematic but workable systems and situations that can be changed and influenced through their choices and actions. For example, Mahatma Gandhi lived within what was to him an unacceptable system—British rule in India—but his situation was such that he had personal power within that system: he was an intelligent lawyer with a passionate temperament and deeply held values of justice. Much of Gandhi's success originated from his internal sense of responsibility and dedication, but we cannot ignore the fact that his position of personal power as a respected lawyer provided possibilities not available to others in India at the time.

So while I am urging you to take responsibility for your choices and actions, I recognize that you may have situations and systems in your life that impair your ability to always make MOGO decisions. At the same time, to whatever degree you are able and given your constraints, you are responsible not only for making MOGO choices in everyday life but also for helping to create MOGO situations and systems.

Responsibility can sound so heavy and dull, even exhausting, but it needn't feel like that. Instead, responsibility can be empowering, energizing, and freeing. When we take on the mantle of responsibility, we are no longer victims of whatever we may feel is victimizing us: corporations, government, advertisers, peer pressures, or social expectations. Instead we become creators of a better life for ourselves and a better world for all.

As Dr. Milgram's and Dr. Zimbardo's experiments revealed, we are often good at rationalizing our decisions and placing blame on someone else, adept at finding excuses for our choices that cause pain and suffering to others. I've often wondered whether the people in Dr. Milgram's experiments later struggled with the knowledge of what they had so willingly done (even though they weren't shocking anyone in reality), and if many changed because of what they learned about themselves. Eighty-four percent of former participants in Dr. Milgram's experiments who were surveyed afterward said they were "glad" or "very glad" to have participated, while 15 percent chose "neutral" (with 92 percent of all former participants responding). Were they glad because of the opportunity that Dr. Milgram provided them—the opportunity to take responsibility for their own actions in the future? One former participant wrote this:

> While I was a subject [participant] in 1964, even though I believed that I was hurting someone, I was totally unaware of why I was doing so. Few people ever realize when they are acting according to their own beliefs and when they are meekly submitting to authority.... To permit myself to be drafted with the understanding that I am submitting to authority's demand to do something very wrong would make me frightened of myself.... I am fully prepared to go to jail if I am not granted Conscientious Objector status. Indeed, it is the only course I could take to be faithful to what I believe."[18]

Obviously, participating in Dr. Milgram's experiment had a profound effect on this man, but we need not have such an extreme experience to be prodded into living according to our values. We can take responsibility for our actions right now.

---

18. See http://www.en.wikipedia.org/wiki/Milgram_experiment.

As the aphorism goes: to whom much is given, much is expected. To the extent to which you are in the enviable position to make decisions about your work, your life, and your family; to make consumer choices; to travel; to communicate freely; to participate in democracy; and to expand your knowledge, the gift and mantle of responsibility is all the greater. So, too, is the joy that comes when you do take responsibility and make your life a reflection of your values. As conservationist and former Pennsylvania governor Gifford Pinchot wrote, "The vast possibilities of our great future will become realities only if we make ourselves responsible for that future."[19]

In the coming chapters, I'll lay the mantle of responsibility on corporations and governments more explicitly, but in the context of this chapter, let us not simply blame multinational corporations, other people's greed, politicians, or any other group. To do so gives away the power we have as individuals to take responsibility for creating the world we long for. While there is no doubt that those in power need to shoulder responsibility, there is also no doubt that each of us must compel them to do so by exercising our own individual power and responsibility to the best of *our* ability.

Practical Suggestions for Embracing Responsibility

➷ Pay attention to your thoughts and language, and notice if you are using words and phrases that place blame on others, deflecting responsibility from yourself. If you find yourself thinking or saying, "So and so did such and such to me," or "If only _____ would stop _____," or "Everything would be fine if _____," try reframing the situation to become aware that you are responsible for your responses and your choices. Meditation teacher Eknath Easwaran reminded people that no one irritates another; rather, people allow themselves to be irritated. As soon as you find yourself ready to blame another, look inward.

---

19. Carl Frankel, *Out of the Labyrinth* (Rhinebeck, NY: Monkfish Book Publishing, 2004), 27.

How can you take responsibility for your own joy and live according to your own values?

- Acknowledge that you choose your actions. Nobody determines how you will act other than you. With this awareness you can make conscious choices and thereby accept responsibility for what you say and do.

- Remember to take responsibility for your attitude. For many months, while writing this book, I was largely incapacitated with sciatica nerve pain. Normally, I can get rather whiny when I'm sick or injured, but this time I was struck by the realization that I still had the capacity to experience joy and contribute to the world in spite of my discomfort. In fact, my appreciation for my laptop grew exponentially during those months because I was able to continue working on this book from my prone position on the couch. I realized that I still bore responsibility for my life and its effects, regardless of my personal situation.

Key 7—Strive for Balance

If I imagine myself reading the first six keys, drawn to this book by the promise of inner peace and a peaceful world but fairly new to the ideas in these pages, I suspect I might feel somewhat overwhelmed about all I've been asked to do, unsure about proceeding to the actual specifics that are coming in part II. So now it is time shift to **Key 7** and focus on balancing your own needs with those of other people, animals, and the environment.

If you think back to the profile of Melissa Feldman in **Key 1— Live Your Epitaph**, you may recall that she referred to the emergency instructions airlines give us when we fly: put an oxygen mask over our own mouth first, then assist our child or others. Airlines tell us to do this because if we do not put our mask on first, we won't be able to help anyone else. The same is true for choosing MOGO. Unless we take care of ourselves we will not be especially helpful to others. With that said, striving for balance does not mean you let yourself off the hook when you face challenges in making MOGO choices. Instead, it means recognizing that your emotional, physical, and spiritual needs are part of the equation, and that striving for balance is integral to creating a MOGO life.

When I think back to my acquisition of knowledge and process of adopting the principle "most good, least harm," I'm well aware that for me it happened very slowly. No one asked me to make connections between all forms of oppression, to model my message and work for change, to take full responsibility for the far-reaching effects of my everyday choices, and then choose the most compassionate products, foods, lifestyle, home, transportation, recreation, and work—starting right now! For almost thirty years I've read books and articles, and watched films on the many issues discussed in this book. Here and there an author or filmmaker has called upon me as a reader or viewer to make a change but not to change every aspect of my life.

Had someone attempted to do what I am now attempting to do with this book, I do not know if I would have been receptive. I like to think so, but I have never been asked to learn about so much so fast, and to make so many different choices. I might have felt overwhelmed and slipped quickly into denial. Or perhaps I would have jumped in, changed everything, and then started proselytizing. Quite possibly, I would have driven everyone around me (and myself) crazy. In fact, despite my slow acquisition of knowledge, I still expected everyone to keep up with me. With every new atrocity I learned about, I was eager to tell others what they should and shouldn't do to make a difference. (And here I am, still doing it!)

I don't want you to dive into MOGO living in such a way that you damage your relationships, or feel overwhelmed or discouraged; that wouldn't be MOGO. What I want so much is for you to be empowered and inspired, and to empower and inspire others. I want you to feel welcomed onto this wonderful path and enthusiastically engaged in the peaceful unfolding of your life and the world.

Although I haven't yet gone into the specific choices that I'll discuss in part II, I've already asked you to take responsibility for so much. I may have promised that it will bring you inner peace and joy, but peace and joy will come from your actions and experiences, and not simply from the intellectual process of reading a book such as this.

My goal is to provide you with enough information and inspiration so that as you embark on the MOGO journey you will find it rewarding, satisfying, and freeing, and the process will bring you the inner peace and joy that you long for.

As I mentioned in the introduction, for the past dozen years I have been training others to be humane educators through a distance learning Master of Education degree and a Humane Education Certificate Program at the Institute for Humane Education. For many of our students, the initial experience is surprisingly internal. They enroll to learn how to teach about the interconnections between human rights, environmental preservation, animal protection, and cultural issues, and to inspire people to be enthusiastic citizens participating in the creation of better world. But before they can educate others about living humanely, they must go on the journey themselves. Many are surprised by the soul-searching they undergo in their effort to best model their message as a teacher. They sometimes feel weighed down with the information, even though their goal is to become someone who will create positive change through education.

These students have our support: the faculty are available at any time; they have a twenty-four-hour online discussion forum with which to communicate with their classmates; they attend a residency week that creates a community of fellow students; and they have two years to complete their course of study. In the online forum, they share stories about difficult challenges—in classrooms as well as with parents, in-laws, friends, and partners—and ask each other how they would handle tricky situations. They give and receive advice, and help each other be more accepting and less judgmental of both themselves and others. Because of the support they have, they are usually able to create healthy balance.

You, however, are probably reading this book alone, learning all these things in the course of days or weeks. Since you may not currently have access to a community of people learning about the issues in this book and making choices accordingly, and may not yet have found a friend or family member to join you in reading and thinking about these issues, I thought it might be helpful to hear from some of our students and graduates. Their experiences will give you ideas about striving for balance in the process of learning and changing so that you can avoid common pitfalls.

Marsha Rakestraw, a graduate of our Humane Education Certificate Program, grew up in a conservative, small town in Kansas. When she went to college she began to learn about issues that had been, until then, completely foreign to her. Together with her husband, she subscribed to an environmental journal, and they later saw a newsletter from an animal protection organization that opened their eyes to animal suffering. As they learned about different issues, they started making changes, such as buying cruelty-free products and making their own household cleaners. Then they stumbled upon the concept of voluntary simplicity and purged their home of excess stuff—something Marsha describes as truly liberating.

Today, Marsha and her husband live in a small condo in a co-housing community. They often use public transit or walk rather than drive. They buy mostly fair trade, organic, and sweatshop-free products, purchasing only what they need and a few luxuries that they really want. They pay attention to the impact of their choices, asking: Does this cause suffering, harm, or destruction to others? Do we really need this thing? What will happen to it when we're done with it?

This is how Marsha describes the process: "It has been like continually updating our eyeglass prescriptions—each time they change, we see a bit more clearly."

I love this metaphor. Marsha is not suggesting that people get an eyeglass prescription that is too strong too soon. Rather, she is suggesting that we update our prescriptions when we are ready. The knowledge we gain when we see more clearly leads to new changes and transformations, but it is knowledge that we are prepared to experience. By proceeding by degrees, we maintain balance.

She goes on to say:

Making the changes in our lives hasn't always been easy. Our families view us with some bewilderment, though with growing acceptance. People often express concern to us about deprivation and making sacrifices, asking, "How could you give up X? How can you live without Y?"

It can be tempting to give in to the "I'm-just-one-person-what-can-I-do?" mantra that our culture feeds us. But even with the struggle and weariness of looking through a lens that sees pain and destruction, I have never felt more powerful. My life is meaningful, joyful, and full of choices that support and nurture a better world.

I've found that the choices I'm making have opened up a world of possibilities. I'm much more creative, a bigger risk taker, more aware of the interconnectedness of everything. There are so many more choices available to me because I'm the one in control of those choices, not some cultural imperative or enticing advertisement. I've discovered so much more abundance and peace in the way I live now.

Marsha's story makes me smile. Many times, I, too, have been asked, "Don't you miss ____?" Or, "You can't eat that, can you? Poor you!" These questions and comments reflect the belief that sacrificing pleasure is always a negative thing, resulting in a sense of deprivation. From the outside looking in, it makes sense that this is how it appears. But from the inside, it is quite different. Marsha's words echo my own experience—greater freedom, joy, and peace come with choosing from our heart and mind, and living according to our values.

We do not mind the word "sacrifice" when it applies to a greater good. We speak of sacrifice for our children, for our elderly parents, or for ideals like freedom and justice. But those who do the everyday sacrificing—whether famous humanitarians such as Mother Teresa or ordinary mothers and fathers—do not think of what they do as sacrifice. What they do comes from love, compassion, commitment, wisdom, and integrity, and in return, feeds them profoundly.

If we begin to feel like we are sacrificing, chances are that our balance is askew, and our task is to find the balance anew. When we get the balance right, we rarely feel that we are sacrificing anything. Chances are, we feel greater inner peace. But if instead of striving for balance when we encounter challenges, we choose to give up on the MOGO principle, I believe that we diminish our lives profoundly, succumbing to what is habitual but not necessarily healthy; what is seemingly easy but not transforming or enlivening.

Even though feelings of sacrifice and deprivation generally disappear once one is on the MOGO path, the fear of these potential emotions can represent a significant obstacle. We may worry that we will be isolated, different, and no longer belong—that the balance will shift away from joy and community. Bob Schwalb, a former computer specialist who graduated from our M.Ed. program in 2005, and who is now a full-time humane educator in Chicago, wrote me the following:

> For me, contemplating changes was actually more difficult than making them. Perhaps I was afraid of the inconvenience. Perhaps I was afraid of failing. Or maybe I was afraid of what others might think. Whatever the reasons, they were real obstacles. These obstacles appeared quite large in the beginning, but they shrank as I realized the changes were really not that inconvenient, that they were not that difficult to follow through on, and that others didn't actually think I was crazy. Armed with this knowledge and confidence, changes came rapidly.

Suzanne Martinson, a student in our M.Ed. program, experienced the shift in her life this way:

> I began to question and research things I always took for granted, and to examine things I never even thought about. Who made this? How was it made? What materials or living beings were hurt or used to create this? How could it be done differently?

My next shift came when I realized that I couldn't rely on someone else to make the changes I felt were important. I needed to participate and no longer felt comfortable being an observer. And as a mother of two small children, this inner drive took on even more meaning, as I would be a role model for future generations.

What is Suzanne's advice to others embarking upon this path?

People don't need to completely overhaul their entire lives if they choose to live a more humane life. They can make small but very meaningful choices. And when there are no choices, seek them out. Nowhere is the concept of supply and demand more relevant.

Sometimes, making personal changes to lead a more MOGO life is not a significant challenge, but interacting positively with others who haven't initiated such changes can be. Judging others and demanding that they change in the ways we want and expect is a common pitfall, also requiring balance.

Roberto Giannicola, a graduate of our Humane Education Certificate Program, is one of those warm, charismatic people to whom others are naturally drawn. He grew up in Italy and Switzerland, and now lives in the United States with his wife and daughter. He is funny, loving, and outgoing. But when he learned about the various issues described in this book and discovered it was not hard to make MOGO choices, he began criticizing others who were not so diligent. Here's how he describes it:

I got angry and wanted to scream at everyone for not making the changes I made. Deciding to make personal changes did require some adjustments, but the main struggles came with the confrontations I had with my friends and family. I had believed that after telling them about what I learned, they would immediately feel the same way, be as shocked as I, and make changes in line with mine. Instead, I was often received with staunch opposition. I fought back, got angry, raised my voice to try to connect them to the issues, but I was only increasing my frustration and not coming to any constructive resolution.

I learned that I cannot go into my friends' houses and bluntly tell them about how destructive their current lifestyle is. Instead, I now teach by example. This has triggered more open discussions with my friends, who are curious and ask me questions. Answering their questions allows me to explain the choices I make based on the MOGO principle, and this raises their curiosity even more—which leads to more discussion. I make it a point to help people understand that it is not so hard to make the transitions, and then provide alternatives for them to consider and choose from.

Roberto has recently launched a program called "Provokare."[20] He offers presentations that inspire people to see the impact they have on others and that demonstrate how people can positively change their lifestyle for the benefit of all. He does all of this in a fun, entertaining, and inviting manner.

Bob, Suzanne, and Roberto remind us to make small but meaningful changes, to anticipate that these changes will be easier than we might imagine, to invite and inspire others, and ultimately to strive for balance. Making MOGO your guiding principle in decision making provides plenty of room for balancing your personal, social, and family needs with the goal of helping others and protecting the environment. You don't have to be perfect. In fact you can't be perfect, and demanding perfection of yourself can unwittingly turn you into someone who demands perfection of others, leaving damaged relationships in your wake and taking you further away from inspiring and welcoming others on a journey that is joyful and positive.

Before I fully embraced the breadth of the MOGO principle I was quite judgmental. I judged not only the slave owner and animal abuser (as I mentioned in **Key 4—Model Your Message and**

---

20. See http://www.provokare.com.

Work for Change), but also the person who drove an SUV; voted for the candidate whom I opposed; hired Chemlawn (now named TruGreen) to spray their lawn with pesticides; ate factory-farmed meat, dairy, and eggs; and so on. Instead of recognizing my own struggles and failures to live in accordance with my values, I judged others' failures. But once I realized the challenge of fully living according to the principle "most good, least harm," I was so much more open to hearing others' interpretations of how to do this.

When I understood that my own annual plane trips caused more carbon dioxide to be released into the atmosphere than my neighbor's SUV; when I came to realize that my vegan diet, though humane to farm animals, might not be as sustainable as a diet derived entirely from local foods; when my son became school-aged and I began to make choices so he would not appear any more different than our family's lifestyle already made him (even though these choices sometimes conflicted with other deeply held values), my judgments of others slowly but surely began to diminish. I was able to start repairing and actively building new bridges. This does not mean that I have turned off my capacity for judgment. We need our good judgment to make MOGO choices. It simply means that I endeavor not to be judgmental.

You are not alone. There are many other people on this journey, too. They are not out to judge you for your failures to live as compassionately and sustainably as possible, just as they hope you will not judge them for their lapses. When you choose not to judge others, you give yourself room not to judge yourself. Then you are free to simply assess the choices before you and make better choices as you are able.

When I lead workshops, I often share the following parable of two fires:

Imagine a campfire in a clearing in the woods. The glow of the fire draws you to it, and its warmth keeps you close. Others are also drawn around the fire, and a wide circle forms, each person full of joy as they are bathed in the warm light.

And now imagine a forest fire raging in those same woods. You and all those around you flee in terror, choking on the smoke, breathless as you try desperately to escape.

Each person has a fire inside them—a fire of passion, commitment, desire, and hope. How well we share this fire with others will determine how readily our fire will ignite a positive revolution toward a better future. If we are like a campfire, we will find ourselves surrounded by others who relish our light and warmth, and follow suit. If we are like a forest fire, we will leave little in our path other than scorched ground with none nearby to listen or share.

Where does the campfire end and the forest fire begin? Usually the forest fire starts with an unexpected wind or spark, when too much fuel is added too quickly and necessary care is not taken.

As you learn about the ways in which your life causes harm and suffering to others, you will be adding fuel to your fire. And you will need to add this fuel carefully and deliberately so that it transforms into warmth and light (the new and positive choices you will make, and the ways in which you will positively influence others) in just the right proportion to glow brightly, rather than consume everyone and everything in sight with your passion, fury, or sorrow.

There is no simple guideline for this. You will have to find your own way, but perhaps if you allow the metaphor of a campfire to capture your imagination, you will have an image to follow. You will know quickly if your campfire is burning too brightly because people will back away from you. And you can pay attention to whether it is burning brightly enough, adding fuel so you can bring some more light into the world and make a greater difference. Strive to find the right balance.

Practical Tools for Striving for Balance

- Take care of yourself. Eat healthy (and humane) foods, exercise regularly, seek out the company of friends, and pursue what brings you the deepest joy.
- Avoid approaching life changes like a crash diet. Instead, make manageable and sustainable changes that can become permanently integrated into your life. Enjoy these changes! Then, when you are ready, make another change. Appreciate each step that you take.

- Brainstorm ideas for a better future. Rather than simply create a list of personal "dos and don'ts," explore your vision for a peaceful world, and identify the most compelling, effective ways that you can help bring about this vision.
- Create a discussion group, a MOGO salon or club, and/or a film series so that you can learn with others how best to put your ethics into practice in a balanced, healthy way. If you have trouble finding people to join you, visit meetup.com and conversationcafe.org to become involved with or to start a discussion or action group near you.

PART II
CHOOSING OUTWARD

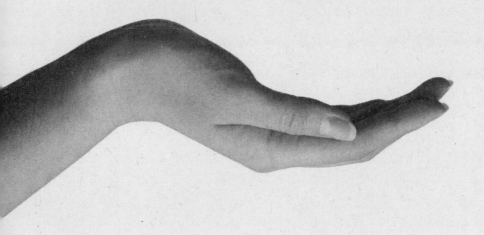

A s you begin part II, it's my hope that you are curious to know more specifics about MOGO living and that you are enthusiastic about the opportunities to make new choices that manifest MOGO in practical and concrete ways in your life. With the inward resolve and the MOGO keys to fuel this journey, it is now time to look outward at the specific choices we make every day: the products we use, the foods we eat, the work we do, the decisions we make about the ways in which we will use our time and energy, and the manner in which we engage in change-making.

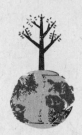

3. Products

We live in the land of products. Our economies revolve around their production and purchase. We are "productophiles." Look around you; put this book down and notice all the products in view. I am going to do the same.

This is what I see:

I am writing in my bedroom. On my desk are two ceramic mugs filled with pens and pencils, a letter opener, a magnifying glass, and scissors. There is my laptop computer and a tray filled to the brim with bills, stamps, papers to file, and papers to read. There is an address book, a date book, a cordless phone, and Post-Its. On the walls are framed paintings, artwork my son has made, and some shelves with objects that have meaning to me—a special shell, a Zuni figurine that was a gift from a friend, a wedding present. To my left is a file cabinet, filled and heavy, and a bookcase with shelves of books, family photos, and six objects that I would classify as knick-knacks. There are two bureaus, stuffed with clothes, and a closet that would take several pages to write about if I were to list everything in it. There's a queen-sized bed with a bunch of pillows, and a dog bed for the dogs. There's a nightstand filled with books, a clock, a lamp, a candle, and a wedding photo. There's a wicker chest with extra linens, a comfortable chair for reading, my husband's bookcase (similarly filled), some houseplants, and a sculpture I made. From my bedroom I can glimpse part of the living room, where I see shelving that holds a CD player, receiver, tape deck, turntable, and record albums—probably a couple hundred of them.

I've just touched the surface. What I can't see is the rest of the house, which is not only our home but also the headquarters of the Institute for Humane Education. Every part of it is filled with stuff. And outside the building itself are two cars that travel a combined twenty-five thousand miles each year because we have chosen to live in a rural area.

One part of me knows that the production of products is what has helped create material wealth for hundreds of millions of people and enabled far more to take small steps out of intolerable poverty. Another part of me knows that each and every product in my home has a story. If I traced the effects of each product, most of the time I would find parts of the story very disturbing indeed. There would be stories of children working long hours in factories instead of going to school and sharing in the opportunities available to my son. There would be the dioxins (a side effect of paper bleaching) that have been force-fed to animals in labs in quantities that kill, and the human health and environmental problems caused by these same dioxins in the ecosystem. There would be many stories of deforestation, resource depletion, and pollution.

There are a few objects that I can look at without the sting of my less-than-humane choices. There's a perfectly formed pine cone that my son gave me, which he found when we were hiking in the woods, a couple of rocks we carried up from the beach, and two beautifully carved pine sticks that my husband made for me. But I suppose I must also consider the knife that he used for carving and tell its story, too.

Since I've gotten in the habit of imagining what you may be thinking as you read this book, here's another list of possible thoughts you might be having right about now:

> 🖊 For crying out loud, this is what makes us human! We are ingenious at toolmaking, and these products are the epitome of our achievements. Do you want us to go back to the Stone Age? Are you a Luddite?

- You're not serious about dissecting every product we have or buy, are you? That would be ridiculous!
- There's no way I'm going to think about the "story" behind every product I use or get.
- If we didn't buy these products, the economies of many nations would collapse; people would suffer terribly. It is thanks to our consumerist lifestyle that we have the freedoms and choices we have, and I wouldn't trade that for anything.
- The products you mention bring you satisfaction and pleasure, I presume. Is that bad?
- You're a total hypocrite! Why are you writing this book when your own life doesn't reflect your values. How do you have any self-respect?

Of course, you may be thinking none of these things, but they are all thoughts that came to my mind when I wrote down the various objects in my bedroom. So what are our options when it comes to MOGO living in relation to such a broad concept as products? What, in fact, does it mean to choose products that do the most good? We do not have to forego the blessings of industrialization, nor do we have to deprive ourselves of products in order to create a MOGO life, but we can make examined choices about the products we choose to ensure that they are ultimately humane and sustainable.

This is what MOGO products mean to me. They are:

- Humane to other people—produced according to fair labor practices that do not exploit, oppress, and cause suffering to others. They provide good jobs and more prosperity.[1]
- Humane to animals—their production does not cause animals to suffer and die.[2]

---

1. One way to meet part of these criteria is to look for a fair trade logo on products. See http://www.transfairuse.org for more information.

2. One way to meet part of these criteria is to look for the logo that ensures that a product has not been tested on animals: http://www.leapingbunny.org.

- 🍃 Sustainable and/or restorative—their production and disposal can be sustained through available resources without causing destruction to ecosystems, and may actually contribute to ecological repair.
- 🍃 Personally life enhancing—they bring something positive to our own lives and do not become more burdensome things to take care of.

It is so much easier to write four bullet points that describe MOGO products than it is to actually choose such products and become conscious of our consumer habits. The list above is so abstract, so divorced from the actual work it takes to choose wisely and humanely when we make purchases. There is no way that I can detail each product category in our lives and provide a list of the products that are MOGO—and, in fact, each of us will differ in our interpretation of the guidelines above.

What I will do instead is choose a few products that are commonplace and provide a framework for considering how to make choices. The questions below can set the stage for any purchases. Before buying a product, ask yourself these three questions:

1. Is the product I am about to buy a want or a need?
2. If it is a need, how can I make sure that I get the most humane and sustainable version of the product, or work for its development?
3. If it is a want, what are the consequences of this purchase to others (humans, animals, and the earth)? Are these consequences worth it?

By asking oneself these questions, buying things becomes a more conscious and deliberate process. What often happens when people actually assess the product choices they make is they buy less; save and care for more; become less influenced by advertising, media, and trends; live more simply; and describe themselves as more self-aware, self-directed, and peaceful. The high of shopping—which is often dissipated when the bills come in—is replaced with the joy of more free time and more relationship- and service-oriented activities.

For those who enjoy shopping and still want to shop with the same gusto as they did prior to considering whether the products they buy are MOGO, the questions above may simply serve as a new shopping guide, inviting the buyer to become a sleuth who seeks out not just the most desirable product or the one at the best price, but rather the product that does the most good. Since I know people who do this, I can attest to the pleasure they derive from finding something they want that does not harm others.

Let's say that you need something to clean your teeth. How will you make the choice about what tooth cleaner, toothbrush, and floss to use? You could use what you have always used and think no more about it, or you could apply the guidelines above to your decision. You might want to know:

1. If the company is known for fair labor practices at home and abroad
2. If the company tests its products on animals or uses only humane, nonanimal tests
3. If the company strives to be environmentally friendly

How can you find the answers to these questions? If you visit responsibleshopper.org and type in the name of your toothpaste (or the company that produces it), you'll quickly learn quite a bit about the company's policies and records, both good and bad. You'll find out if there are any campaigns against the company, and also if it has received any kudos.[3] You can do this research with virtually every well-known company, whether it produces toothpaste and other personal care products, clothes, drugs, housewares, cars, appliances, cosmetics, and so on.

In the case of toothpaste, your choices may come down to the following:

---

3. While http://www.responsibleshopper.org does not list every company, it does have information about most of the larger companies and their products.

- A reasonably priced, well-known toothpaste produced by a big company that tests on animals, uses ingredients and packaging from foreign sources that do not protect workers, promotes extensive sales of its products in countries where they may replace adequate local versions, constantly produces "new and improved" versions to get you to buy more than you need, has questionable environmental practices, and uses ingredients that may not be healthy
- A more expensive, lesser-known toothpaste by a smaller company that practices more humane and sustainable policies relating to the environment, people, and animals, and which uses healthier ingredients
- Inexpensive baking soda and water made into a paste, reducing packaging, testing, environmental destruction, and cutting cost as well

What you choose depends on your values, preferences, and willingness to learn new information. I never knew that a mixture of baking soda and water was an adequate toothpaste until I was an adult, and I read about this choice in a nonprofit organization's newsletter. Certainly, no one was advertising this option on television.

There's more to cleaning our teeth than the cleaner we use; we also make choices about the toothbrush. Most toothbrushes are discarded after several months, necessitating the purchase of a new one. One of the assignments that the students in our Master of Education and certificate programs must complete is to choose a product and trace its effects from beginning to end. A few years ago, one of the students chose a toothbrush. I was amazed to see an analysis of this simple and ubiquitous product. What was somewhat heartening, after reading about the massive numbers of plastic toothbrushes that are produced and discarded each year, was to learn that there were some companies producing toothbrushes with exchangeable heads so that the entire toothbrush did not need to be discarded. Instead, a new brush head would take the place of the used one—a simple choice that has a small but positive effect. Some companies produce toothbrushes using recycled and recyclable plastic as well. There are also companies that produce floss that comes in recycled paper containers rather than hard plastic—another simple choice that makes a small but collectively bigger impact. If these particular choices aren't available at your local drugstore or supermarket chain, you can either ask that they be stocked (a way to use your voice to help create more change), or visit a natural foods supermarket, a health food store, or a food co-op.

Let's say the product choice you are considering is clothing. I suspect that, like most readers of this book, you have more clothes than you actually need. Yet you may still want, or even feel you need, more. I know that despite a closet full of clothes I still feel like I need a sweater in a certain color (to match a pair of pants I have). I know, of course, that I don't really *need* this, but I still feel like I do, and the pull to satisfy that perceived need is great enough to draw me into stores to take a look. Let's say I decide to satisfy these perceived needs. What choices do I have to make sure that the clothing and shoes I purchase are MOGO?

I could:

- Go to a big-box chain store where the clothing and shoes are inexpensive, but where little—if any—effort is being made to ensure that foreign workers are paid a living wage or are provided with humane working conditions; where local employees face insurmountable obstacles to unionizing; where its sales are negatively affecting the downtown community; and where its practices are known to have a poor environmental record.
- Go to a locally owned store that sells clothes from companies committed to improving the working conditions of factory workers and the environmental impacts of their clothing production (where I will generally pay more than at the cheap, big-box store).
- Buy online from a company that only sells clothes that are organic, produced under fair and healthy working conditions, and not made with materials that come from animals

(where I will also generally pay more than at the chain store).

📌 Visit local thrift shops to avoid participating directly in sweatshop labor and to recycle discarded clothes (and also save a lot of money).

📌 Trade clothes with friends at a clothing swap (which is free!).

These are some of the decisions we are each faced with when we buy clothes, although the issues are far more complex than these four choices indicate. For example, if we do decide to buy new clothes but our budget constrains us to shop at a cheap big-box chain, we could still work for change through letter-writing campaigns and public education about the company's inhumane policies. This same company that may be exploiting or discriminating against workers, destroying downtown centers, creating traffic problems, and polluting local waterways might also be providing donations to local causes in our community, or its valuable stock might be ensuring some people decent pensions when they retire.

While we can acknowledge the good that such companies may do, this does not mean that we ought to absolve them of responsibility for the harm they cause or the exploitation they perpetrate. We can applaud their occasional good corporate citizenship while working to influence them to do much more.[4]

You might think your voice is not that powerful and that you don't really have the ability to influence systemic change, but that's simply not true. Because of citizen efforts in San Francisco, for example, it is now illegal for the city's tax dollars to support sweatshops. Since 2005, San Francisco's firefighters' uniforms, computers, hospital food, and more have been produced through fair labor standards that ensure living wages and safe working conditions for employees. This groundbreaking legislation continues to lead the way for more such legislation in other cities. You can be part of making your community sweatshop-free, too.[5]

---

4. For an illuminating and powerful exposé of the world's biggest company, you can watch the 2005 film *Wal-Mart: The High Cost of Low Price*.

5. See http://www.sweatfree.org.

Of course, we shouldn't stop making connections at this point. Fair wages and good working environments, while a fantastic advance, are not the only goal. If the computers produced under good labor standards are still being manufactured with minerals mined through destructive practices, using toxic chemicals that create dangerous disposal problems, and if the foods served in hospital cafeterias are the products of animal cruelty and are nonorganic, then we haven't gone far enough in envisioning and creating products that are MOGO. We can celebrate wonderful victories without becoming complacent.

There are so many choices we make that can affect others. A rug may come from a company where children worked as slaves, hand-tying each knot, or it may come from a company committed to humane treatment of workers and fair wages.[6] Your chocolate bar may come from a corporation that purchases cocoa from sellers who rely upon child and slave labor to gather the beans, or your chocolate may come from a company that produces chocolate from fairly traded, organic cocoa beans.[7] The diapers you buy can be the plastic, disposable variety, filled with chemicals, or they can be more ecological, biodegradable disposables (available at natural foods supermarkets and co-ops). Or you can choose cloth diapers that you launder and reuse, preventing more plastic production and more accumulation of solid waste.

Even the most ubiquitous choices have an impact. Take the common can of soda: from the energy-intensive and polluting bauxite mining to make the aluminum; the toxic chemicals in the paint on the can; the effects on societies where bottling plants not only dry up dwindling supplies of community water but also pollute the existing water; the significant fossil fuels needed to transport liquids; the energy used for refrigeration to cool the sodas; the disposal challenges and failures to recycle; and the personal health and dental effects of drinking the soda, there is much to consider before deciding to put your money in a vending machine.

---

6. Look for the RugMark label on imported rugs. This label ensures that the rug was produced through fair labor: http://www.rugmark.org.

7. See http://www.stopchildlabor.org.

Unfortunately, the current trend in bottled water is only marginally better. The health consequences of drinking water over soda are obviously positive, but bottled water creates the same environmental problems as bottled soda, simply to profit on a product that is, in many parts of the world, provided free or at low cost through a tap or well. The explosion of bottled water is one of those trends that demonstrate how easily advertising influences us to adopt behaviors and beliefs. We have been convinced to spend more money per gallon of bottled water than per gallon of gasoline! (With rising prices this ratio is changing, but you get the picture.) Below are some of the consequences of the 28 billion bottles of water that are purchased in the United States alone:

- Eight percent wind up in landfills; only 20 percent are recycled.[8]
- Making the plastic bottles requires 17 million barrels of oil per year.[9]
- Production of bottled water in 2006 resulted in 2.5 million tons of carbon dioxide emissions.[10]
- For Fiji water, 250 grams of carbon dioxide are released for every bottle produced (93 grams to produce the bottle in China; 4 grams to transport the empty bottle to Fiji; 153 grams to transport the full bottle from Fiji to the United States).[11]
- The average energy cost for a bottle of water (including the production of the bottle, transportation, and disposal) is equivalent to "filling up a quarter of every bottle with oil."[12]

---

8. These statistics come from http://www.pacinst.org/topics/water_and_sustainability/ bottled_water_and_energy.html.

9. Ibid.

10. Ibid.

11. These statistics come from http://www.treehugger.com/files/2007/02/pablo_calculate.php.

12. These statistics come from http://www.pacinst.org/topics/water_and_sustainability/ bottled_water_and_energy.html.

- It takes 3 to 5 liters of water to produce a single liter of bottled water. In the case of imported water, like Fiji, it takes 6.74 liters.[13]
- Dasani from the Coca-Cola Company and Aquafina from Pepsi-Cola are simply purified tap water.[14]
- Twenty-five percent of bottled waters are simply reprocessed municipal waters.[15]
- Twenty-two percent of brands that were tested contain, in at least one sample, chemical contaminants at levels above strict state health limits.[16]
- The plastic containers may leak hazardous chemicals such as phthalates into the water.[17]

If one is concerned about chemicals in tap water, or heavy metals and bacteria in well water, it's easy enough to install a countertop water filter, a far less expensive measure, both personally and environmentally, than buying bottled water. San Francisco has led the way on this issue, too. Because of citizen efforts, the mayor issued an executive order in 2007 banning the purchase of bottled water with tax dollars. Seattle, Washington, followed suit in 2008.

There are times when bottled water is a necessity. In areas where ground water is polluted, during droughts, and when electricity fails, bottled water is a lifesaver, but we do not need vending machines selling bottled water next to water fountains, and we do not need to drink bottled water when we have access to perfectly adequate tap water. If we want ready access to water, we can simply fill a stainless steel water bottle or canteen and carry it with us.

13. These statistics come from http://www.treehugger.com/files/2007/02/pablo_calculate.php.

14. These statistics come from http://www.cnn.com/2007/HEALTH/07/27/pepsico.aquafina.reut/.

15. These statistics come from http://www.trygoodwater.com/what_about_plastic.htm.

16. These statistics come from http://www.nrdc.org/water/drinking/qbw.asp.

17. These statistics come from http://www.trygoodwater.com/what_about_plastic.htm.

If we begin to look at all of our purchases—even the most mundane like those mentioned above—through the MOGO lens, we inevitably begin to make MOGO product choices. We can also begin to envision and then invest in the production of products that offer better choices so that we won't be in the uninspiring position of weighing the bottled beverage and our desire to drink it against the earth and its inhabitants. Imagine a container for beverages that is made of a biodegradable nutrient. Where I live, apple trees are abundant. Perhaps one day local cider will be pressed into containers that can be composted and dug back into people's gardens when the cider is finished. Currently, there are companies producing such biodegradable plastics for bottling water, some that include built-in filters, and one day "bio-plastics" may be the norm for packaging.

Most of us in industrialized countries consume enormous quantities of fossil fuels. Between home heating oil, automobiles, and trips on planes, our high-consumption, mobile lifestyles are drying up oil wells. We fight wars over oil, and we despoil the earth and its oceans with oil spills. We pollute the air and contribute to global climate change by burning coal and fossil fuels. With awareness and commitment, however, we can reduce our use of these fuels by choosing different products and lifestyles. We can also move far more quickly to create model societies that are not oil dependent.

Many companies are working toward transforming our energy economy, even some of the big multinationals that have been notorious for pollution and excessive resource consumption in the past. By supporting such companies in their transformation, we can contribute to a more rapid, responsible change. There's a difference between blindly accepting corporate greenwashing, in which the biggest polluters try to persuade us that they are now "green," and supporting those corporations making the shift toward responsible and sustainable production.

Whether or not General Electric and Ford Motor Company (as two examples) are sincere in their commitment to invent sustainable products and systems—as their CEOs have stated—is yet to be seen, but our diligence in holding these corporations accountable may make the difference between catastrophe and innovative, timely, healthy change.[18] We can take on a threefold responsibility using the 3 *Vs*: (1) Voice our concerns through letters, emails, and blogs, and by participating in existing campaigns so that we have a greater impact; (2) Vote for candidates who will commit to holding corporations accountable for the harm they cause; and (3) withhold support from companies whose policies and actions are destructive or inhumane by using our monetary Veto, and support those companies striving to make MOGO products (see chapter 6, **Activism, Volunteerism, Democracy**).

Back to oil: one of the most obvious product choices to discuss in the context of fossil fuels is the automobile. Because of the growing demand for and commitment to fuel efficiency, by the time this book is published there will be more options for environmentally friendlier, fuel-efficient, or perhaps even hydrogen-fueled vehicles. Although I don't believe that fuel efficiency is the answer to the problems caused by burning oil, it is a critical first step to slowing destruction while we seek out real change. There is finally a significant effort among some oil companies and auto manufacturers to address the decline in world petroleum reserves as well as global warming. If, as McDonough and Braungart suggest in their book, *Cradle to Cradle*, we envision something that's not simply less bad but which is quite good, we can create a future in which vehicles are fully recyclable and run on renewable, nonpolluting fuel, and whose exhaust and tire dust are biological nutrients. In this way, we

---

18. So, too, it is crucial that we be diligent in seeing beyond the hype of companies that may do some good, but do far more harm. For example, Philip Morris, the well-known tobacco company, transformed its image dramatically in recent years. First, it renamed itself Altria. The word Altria might make us think "altruistic," which the company is decidedly not since tobacco products literally kill millions. Altria's full-page ads in popular magazines would have us believe that the company is in fact altruistic, since the ads talk about solving domestic violence and other social problems. Altria owns many of the best-known food companies, including Kraft foods. This means that many of us unwittingly support a tobacco company when we shop for food.

will not only slow the pace of environmental destruction and potential economic decline, we will actually create a healthy, economically thriving society.

Depending upon where you live, you may or may not require an automobile. If you live in Manhattan, you probably don't need to own a car, but if you live, as I do, in a rural area, you most likely do. Advertising will try to convince you that you need an SUV, the bigger the better, and you will have to weigh your desires against the future for generations to come, human and nonhuman. Until we have shifted to a nonpolluting and nutrient-producing transportation economy, we each can take responsibility for slowing the process of environmental degradation. There are many ways to do this. You can:

- Choose the most fuel-efficient vehicle that meets your needs, if you must rely on a car.
- Join a car sharing group such as zipcar (zipcar.com) if you sometimes need a car.
- Carpool as much as possible and join a ridesharing group such as GoLoco (goloco.org), which allows you to carpool almost anywhere, anytime.
- Take public transportation as much as you can.
- Ride a bike and get exercise while you travel.

It's important not to stop here, however. Pressure both on companies as well as elected officials to invest in clean energy is paramount, and creating a climate that quickens our commitment to real innovation is essential.

I realize that the list of things I'm asking you to do is growing longer and longer, but I can tell you that when people make these choices, they generally feel better in a variety of ways. Those who join GoLoco get to meet people and make new friends through car sharing. Those who begin biking become more fit. Those who take public transportation sometimes meet people who become important in their lives (like Melissa, described in the first section of this book, did on the subway).

It's a good idea to take an inventory of your energy usage and calculate your personal contribution to the problems caused by burning fossil fuels. Once you know, you are in a better position to evaluate your choices. Several organizations and websites can help you. For example, myfootprint.org calculates your ecological footprint by asking you questions and analyzing your answers. After completing this inventory, you'll have more information to lower your ecological footprint score. There are obvious and simple choices—turning off lights and replacing incandescent bulbs with compact fluorescents, not letting water run unnecessarily, lowering the thermostat when it's cold and raising the temperature for air conditioning when it's hot, eating primarily plant-based and locally produced foods (see the next chapter), along with the other ideas mentioned in relation to transportation above.

Then there are bigger purchase items that have larger consequences. Unless you live in a wind- or solar-powered building, the size of your home and its insulation, along with the appliances you choose, make a huge difference in fossil fuel use. Although family size is not growing, individual homes are getting bigger and bigger, requiring more and more energy to build, heat, and cool. Choosing a smaller home and energy-efficient appliances saves significant amounts of fuel and money. But again, McDonough and Braungart offer us an even better vision. They are designing buildings that work with the existing climate and topography, including rooftop gardens, wastewater treatment through biological mechanisms, and nutrient-generating systems. These are the exciting ventures that you can become part of, while in the meantime choosing the best options currently available to you.

There are countless home-oriented choices that impact other people, animals, and the environment. From the paint, flooring, carpeting, and furniture to the building materials themselves, we are affecting many others through our choices, potentially adversely. Toxins abound in many conventional homebuilding and furnishing products, from PVC (vinyl) to formaldehyde. But there are alternatives to most of the toxic products on the market. You can visit the healthy building network (healthybuilding.net) for tips on making your home less toxic, and you can also check out other organizations and websites listed in chapter 12, **Recommended Resources**.

Some of the furniture we buy, especially tropical wood furniture like teak and mahogany, may come at the expense of razed rainforests and old-growth trees, but many companies now sell sustainably harvested woods. You can find out where to purchase such furniture from the Forest Stewardship Council, fscus.org. I believe that most of us would prefer to have a coffee table that didn't come at the expense of animals whose habitats are disappearing due to rainforest destruction. When in doubt, there is always the option of buying from an antique shop or used furniture store, thus reusing what currently exists rather than contributing to further resource depletion.

I love giving gifts, but I don't like buying stuff that may be harming other people, other species, or the environment, and I don't like contributing to waste. Each holiday season, I ask myself what I can offer that is fun, aligned with my values, and not too time-consuming to produce. Usually, I find a theme for the year. One year a friend taught me how to make paste paper, a process that is as pleasurable as finger painting was as a child, but which results in more varied and sturdy results. I invited some children to join my son and me, and we spent an afternoon making beautiful paste paper, recycling existing waste paper in the process. Another friend taught us how to make paper boxes, so we used our paste paper to make lovely little boxes as gifts (and to hold gifts of other crafts).

For my birthday a few years ago, a friend of mine made me a jar of memories. She took a tomato sauce container and filled it with slips of paper, each of which described a memory she had of our friendship. It was so much fun to read each piece of paper, and recall the great times and poignant moments we had shared. Other friends have given our family baked treats during the holidays, a perfect gift that never gets thrown out or forgotten but, rather, relished.

One of the traditions in our home is to give coupon gifts. Each year for the past several years I've created a box of promissory gifts for my son, one for each month. One month might be a promise to make his favorite three dinners. Another might be the promise to create a treasure hunt (the treasure usually being found objects or family heirlooms). Still another might be the promise to take him and his friends to a local baseball game. These are the kinds of gifts that make life better, not simply more full of stuff to care for, find space for, and ultimately dispose of.

When you take out the trash, is it a job you enjoy? Would you rather have less trash to dispose of? When you hear a report on a summer day that the air is not healthy to breathe in your region, and when you read in your paper that rates of asthma in children are skyrocketing, do you feel a sense of dis-ease? Our individual choices contribute to such reports, though it is often difficult to see how because we are not encouraged or inspired to imagine living differently—in ways that contribute positively.

The book *Stuff: The Secret Lives of Everyday Things* traces the effects of half a dozen everyday products, giving us a taste of their true costs and reminding us that our product choices have effects beyond our own pleasure and pocketbooks. Reading this short book is sobering, yet it is also fascinating and exciting to know how we impact others. With knowledge comes the power to live more deeply in accordance with our values and more effectively contribute to a better world.

When we choose products that help and forgo products that hurt, we are not only casting a monetary vote; we are collectively installing a new kind of administration—one that values and promotes a MOGO world. Corporations respond to demand. If the demand is for an endless supply of disposable products that quickly turn into landfill or toxic ash through incineration, or that are shipped off to poorer countries for disposal, corporations will produce just that—at the expense of the environment, other people, and animals. If the demand is for recyclable, humane, and ecologically healthy and restorative products produced through fair wages, companies will supply them, and we will all benefit.

We are not used to asking questions when we buy products. It can feel awkward to ask the manager at the store whether the product we're about to buy was made through the exploitation of disenfranchised, desperate people, or the destruction of rainforests, or the pollution of aquifers. There's a good chance the manager won't know. She might be bewildered by such questions or initially offended. While you may feel embarrassed or uncomfortable about broaching these subjects with company employees, think of it this way: you are giving these companies an opportunity to do better, and to serve you and the world. You are also empowering the person you speak with to make MOGO choices, too. You're providing the fuel to ignite a discussion and a vision of a better world through kinder practices and choices. You may be planting the seeds of great ideas. Seen in this way, your choice to spend and speak for change—in a positive, nonjudgmental, respectful, and visionary way that recognizes the need to find solutions that benefit people, animals, and ecosystems simultaneously—can inspire others to do the same, from the custodian, who might start using nontoxic, cruelty-free cleaners, to the CEO, who might make positive changes that improve all aspects of his or her company.

For decades, most corporations have had no choice but to increase their profits for shareholders by every legal means possible. In fact, as Jared Diamond points out in *Collapse*, our laws have made a corporation's directors liable "for something termed 'breach of fiduciary responsibility' if they knowingly manage a company in a way that reduces profits. The car manufacturer, Henry Ford, was successfully sued by stockholders in 1919 for raising the minimum wage of his workers to $5 per day: the court declared that while Ford's humanitarian sentiments about his employees were nice, his business existed to make profits for its stockholders."[19]

Fortunately, these laws are changing. More than forty states have amended their corporate statutes to permit corporate boards to consider workers and the community (sometimes referred to as stakeholders).[20] Unfortunately, these amendments have not yet resulted in significant changes in corporate responsibility.

---

19. Jared Diamond, *Collapse* (New York: Viking, 2005), 483–484.

20. Frances Moore Lappé, *Democracy's Edge* (San Francisco: Jossey-Bass, 2006), 85.

Robert Hinkley wants to change this. A corporate lawyer turned advocate for corporate responsibility, Hinkley realized that without a more significant change in our legal system, the effort to compel corporations to act ethically will always conflict with the corporate mandate to maximize profits. He has created a code of responsibility that, if made into law, will prevent corporations from profit-making at the expense of people and the environment, and enable them to compete successfully in a marketplace in which all other corporations have the same guidelines. His vision lies in twenty-eight words added to each state's corporate statute. According to Hinkley's code of conduct, the corporation will continue to pursue profit, "but not at the expense of the environment, human rights, public health or safety, welfare of the communities in which the corporation operates, or dignity of its employees." While my hope is that these state codes will also prohibit the abuse of animals, I am excited about the potential for such legal measures to revolutionize business practices.

Whether or not Hinkley's code is made into law in different states and countries does not absolve us of responsibility for our individual choices. As Diamond says, we citizens must take responsibility ourselves, not because corporations are blameless but because we effectively create our corporations with our laws and policies, as well as with our checkbooks. He writes:

In the long run, it is the public, either directly or through our politicians, that has the power to make destructive environmental policies unprofitable and illegal, and to make sustainable environmental policies profitable. The public can do that by suing businesses for harming them, as happened after the Exxon Valdez, Piper Alpha, and Bhopal disasters; by preferring to buy sustainably harvested products, a preference that caught the attention of Home Depot and Unilever; by making employees of companies with poor track records feel ashamed of their company and complain to their own management; by preferring their governments to award valuable contracts to businesses with a good environmental track record ... and by pressing their governments to pass and enforce laws and egulations requiring good environmental practices. ...

To me, the conclusion that the public has the ultimate responsibility for the behavior of even the biggest businesses is empowering and hopeful, rather than disappointing. My conclusion is not a moralistic one about who is right or wrong, admirable or selfish, a good guy or a bad guy. My conclusion is instead a prediction, based on what I have seen happening in the past. Businesses have changed when the public came to expect and require different behavior. . . .[21]

It is my hope that this chapter leaves you envisioning the positive effects you might have, rather than feeling like an internal harasser, telling you not to buy something you want, has just taken up residence in your brain. Desire is a complicated emotion. Rarely do we desire one thing in isolation, yet a strong desire can easily eclipse other desires. For example, you might sincerely want a less polluted environment and a reversal of global warming, and you might also want an SUV. You might deeply desire a sustainable, cohousing community in which to live, and you might also want a home with more privacy that does not require group decision-making. You might wish to live more simply, free of advertising's insidious influences, and yet you might also want the products (and the satisfactions promised by those products) that you see advertised all around you.

What if you were to shift the focus of your desires just a bit? What if you opened up yourself to the possibility that you could fulfill your desires even more deeply, resulting in even more satisfaction, without choosing the product that causes harm and without choosing to buy so many products in general? Materialism rarely brings joy or inner peace. Over and over, those who have chosen to reject the consumerist messages of our culture in favor

---

21. Frances Moore Lappé, *Democracy's Edge* (San Francisco: Jossey-Bass, 2006), 484.

of greater simplicity report that their lives improve substantially. They are happier and healthier. Their choices bring them greater peace of mind and contribute to a more sustainable and peaceful world for all. All that you need to allow such shifts to occur is the willingness to learn and explore what else is out there, and what else you can help create.

Practical Suggestions for Choosing Products

Although I've offered many suggestions throughout this chapter, here are just a few closing ideas to consider:

- Pause long enough before you make purchases to assess your options and choose according to your values.
- Before you buy, find out whether the product is made from recycled materials and is recyclable, and determine whether you would be able to repair it if it broke.
- Consider a visit to the library instead of buying books, music, and videos (most libraries now have music and film sections).[22]
- Find out what your neighbors and friends have that you might borrow, and consider what you have that you could share.[23]
- Try making gifts instead of buying them. Making things brings joy to the maker as well as the receiver.

---

22. I realize that this is a strange suggestion coming from someone who would very much like people to buy her books, but if every library had a copy of this, and my other books, I would be quite happy indeed. My own criterion for buying books is based on whether I'll want to revisit the book periodically or use it as a reference.

23. Visit http://www.neighborrow.com.

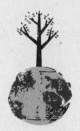

4. Food

F ood choices are among the most personal decisions we
make, and discussions about diet are among the most sensitive. Many of us have very strong opinions about food that stem
from family traditions, religion, culture, what we enjoy eating,
what we have been taught and what we believe about nutrition,
our body image, how certain foods make us feel emotionally
and physically, and, for some people, our ethics.

I would venture to guess that for most people, ethics are not a
primary issue in their dietary choices. Most of us eat what we
were raised to eat, as well as what our culture promotes, adver-
tises, and sells. You may eat few plantains (a relative of the
banana) because you never ate plantains growing up, do not
know how to cook and prepare them, and do not even know
where to buy one. If a plantain salad (similar to potato salad)
were prepared for you at a friend's house, and if you liked it, you
might add plantains to your diet. But you probably wouldn't
question the ethics of eating plantains. We just do not often ask
moral questions about our food.

Yet food choices are among the most important in the quest
for doing the most good and the least harm. Modern agricultural
practices are often destructive, oppressive, cruel, and, for the
most part, hidden. Our individual food choices affect our health,

the environment, other people, and other species. Perhaps more than any other choice we make in our daily lives, diet has the most far-reaching consequences.

If, for example, we were to make connections between a typical food choice and its myriad effects (as was done with the T-shirt in **Key 3—Make Connections and Self-Reflect**), what might we find? Let's look at a fast food hamburger.

The fast food burger is high in fat, salt, cholesterol, and calories, and usually contains pesticides, hormones, and drug residues. Sometimes it contains dangerous (occasionally fatal) bacteria. Eating these burgers in quantity may lead to weight gain, obesity, high blood pressure, strokes, heart disease, various cancers, impotence, type 2 diabetes, osteoporosis, and other health problems.

Such health problems are commonplace in the United States, contributing to health care costs that are skyrocketing, a growing percentage of people without health insurance, increased taxes to pay for the uninsured, fewer raises at work because employer health care costs are gobbling up profits, and more.

Scientists are at work trying to cure many of these largely preventable diseases, to perfect surgical procedures, and to produce new drugs to counteract many of our self-created health problems. In the process, they are killing millions of animals in laboratories. Rabbits, birds, dogs, cats, mice, cows, pigs, sheep, and primates (among others) are drugged, made ill, genetically engineered, cut open, and finally killed when the experiments are over. Meanwhile, medical students entering the profession discover few courses on preventive medicine or nutrition. In a telling *Philadelphia Inquirer* article, the reporter pointed out that preventive medicine doesn't pay back the huge student loans of medical students because people stay healthier and require less medical care.

The fast food hamburger is part of a much larger system that includes the suffering and death of cows and calves, enormous water pollution, significant fossil fuel use, soil erosion, wasted grain, fresh water depletion, rainforest destruction, loss of biodiversity, and greenhouse gas production.

People are exploited in this process as well. Slaughterhouse workers suffer the highest injury rates of any profession in the

United States. Many of these employees are illegal immigrants who have fled their own country's poverty and oppression, and have no health insurance. If they seek medical attention for their injuries—which they may or may not, given their illegal status—they have little money to pay for it.

And the fast food nation (soon to be world) that we have created has contributed to suburban sprawl, more car use (and hence more pollution and climate-altering gases in the air), more traffic accidents, more strip malls, fewer downtown centers, and less community.

And so on.

I've only just touched the surface of the fast food hamburger, not mentioning many of the issues raised in Eric Schlosser's excellent book, *Fast Food Nation*, or in the enlightening film, *Super Size Me*. Yet even in an entire book on the subject of fast food, Schlosser himself fails to mention several of the connections above, making us realize just how many connections there are with something as simple as a burger.[1] When we unlock the door to the most common of our food choices, we see countless interconnected passageways leading to ever more doors. If we view the fast food hamburger in isolation, as a dietary preference or convenience food and nothing more, then we fail to recognize the connections between our choice and its many effects. But when we open the doors of this labyrinth, we create the possibility for not only making better food choices but also solving problems in many of the various "rooms" that are all connected to one another.

There is no single diet that is the most sustainable and humane. Depending upon where you live, and your climate and terrain, a MOGO diet will include a variety of factors. But in general, eating organic and seasonal foods that are produced locally[2] and a

---

1. It's not simply fast food burgers that come with these costs; so do all fast food meals, to greater and lesser degrees, as well as conventional supermarket and restaurant beef, pork, turkey, chicken, dairy products, and eggs.

2. One way to buy local foods is to visit a farmers' market in your area or to patronize a local grocery store that makes it a practice to buy local foods. To find out about regional farmers' markets visit http://www.ams.usda.gov/farmersmarkets.

primarily plant-based[3] whole foods diet, does more good and less harm to you, animals, and the environment than eating animal-based products, processed foods, and pesticide-sprayed (i.e., conventional) produce that has been transported long distances.

When we sit down to eat, unless we have grown, raised, and killed the food in front of us, there is much we do not know. And until we learn about the effects of our food choices, we cannot make the best dietary decisions. Unfortunately, if we are eating the typical American diet, the chances are high that we're consuming foods that contribute to significant environmental destruction, disenfranchisement of farmers, and, in the case of animal-based foods, cruelty.

The issue of animal cruelty in agriculture is rarely discussed in the media. Diet articles and talk shows generally revolve around weight loss or health. Some recent books and films have thankfully begun to explore social justice and environmental issues regarding modern food production, but there is little information in the mainstream media about the animals who wind up on our plates. Thus, the image that most of us have of animals on the farm is from an era that has long since passed. Most still imagine hens pecking outdoors and sitting in their nest boxes to lay their eggs. We still envision pigs in barnyards, rolling around in the cool mud, and cows spending their lives grazing on wide, open fields. But sadly, for over 95 percent of the animals consumed in the United States, such images have nothing at all to do with reality.

I have visited factory farms—those modern facilities that supply the vast majority of meat, dairy products, and eggs to consumers—and I've been shocked by what I have seen, smelled, and heard. Visiting one of the largest egg-producing factories on the East Coast, I saw hundreds of thousands of hens crammed into cages so small they were unable to stretch a wing. I listened to the cries

---

3. The United Nation's Food and Agriculture Organization, cited in "Rethinking the Meat Guzzler," *New York Times*, January 27, 2008, estimates that livestock production, because of a combination of methane waste, inefficient conversion of plants to flesh, and enormous fossil fuel use in production, generates nearly a fifth of the world's greenhouse gases—more than transportation.

of the birds that sounded like screaming. I choked on the fumes from their accumulated wastes, which they had to breathe twenty-four hours a day for the approximately year-long duration of their lives. This facility was not only perfectly legal but also represented the norm for modern commercial egg production.

When I arrived with a group of students for a tour of this particular facility, our guide, a friendly and obviously caring man, proudly showed off this factory that was producing millions of eggs for consumers from Maryland to Maine. But when one of the students asked him if we could see the birds, his face fell.

"Yes, but it's not as nice," he responded.

He did not seem to like the cruelty inherent in the system either.

The birds' beaks had all been sliced in half, without anesthesia, to prevent them from killing each other under such extreme confinement and stress; but even their deformed beaks could do damage, and many of the chickens had open, oozing sores. When the tour brought us to the pharmaceutical room and we learned about the drugs fed to sick animals, we asked how they were able to treat just the sick ones. Clearly, we had asked a silly question: all the birds were routinely fed antibiotics and other drugs in their feed. That's what kept them alive under these conditions.

I have also brought students to see a confinement veal operation, those infamous factories where male calves of dairy cows are chained at the neck in tiny stalls, unable to take more than one step forward or backward.[4] If we wish to make MOGO food choices, it's important to know the reality behind what we eat, and, for example, inquire about the conditions under which these poor calves live before they are killed at four months old, anemic to keep their flesh pale, with atrophied muscles to keep their flesh tender.

Pigs fare no better than these calves, nor are turkeys exempt from de-beaking and confinement. Dairy cows must endure the sorrow of their young taken away at a day old, and some bellow

---

4. Dairy cows are impregnated annually so that they will continually produce milk. Their male offspring are of no use to the dairy industry, so they often wind up as veal.

out for days when for all intents and purposes their newborns are kidnapped. Surely, the fact that half of U.S. dairy cows wind up suffering from mastitis, a painful udder infection, speaks to a system gone awry.

And what about fish? While fish are often touted as health food, the carnivorous fishes humans consume concentrate the toxins and pollutants that we dump into our waterways up the food chain, making their flesh repositories of mercury, PCBs, and other poisonous substances. Regulatory agencies advise women of childbearing years, as well as children, to eat minimal amounts of fish, lest they consume toxic levels of these pollutants. The trend toward aquaculture (fish "farming") often exacerbates this problem, with "farm"-raised fishes being some of the most unhealthy to eat, and their wastes contaminating and polluting bays.

Even if the flesh of fishes were not so polluted, there are ethical considerations involved in their consumption as well. The oceans are literally being strip-mined, with mile-long nets scouring the seas and killing everything in their path—by some estimates including about a thousand marine mammals per day[5] along with millions of nontarget sea animals. Aquaculture does not prevent overfishing since, on average, three pounds of wild fish are caught and fed to the penned fish in order to produce every one pound that is "farm" raised, depleting species that had previously been ignored by the industry.[6] One fishery after another is collapsing, often permanently.[7] And what is rarely discussed or considered is the suffering the fish endure—slow death by suffocation or long-line hooks that drag fishes by their sensitive mouths for hours before they are killed. An estimated two billion long-line hooks are set worldwide each year, each line baited with up to ten thousand hooks. Not only do long-lines kill their intended prey (primarily tuna and swordfish) but also approximately forty

---

5. See http://www.cetaceanbycatch.org.

6. Julia Whitty, "The Fate of The Ocean," *Mother Jones* (March/April 2006): 37.

7. Evidence shows, however, that if we stop or diminish fishing in certain areas, most fish species recover.

thousand sea turtles, three hundred thousand seabirds, and millions of sharks annually.[8]

In chapter 11, **Relevant Facts and Statistics**, you'll find statistics related to the effects of animal agriculture on the environment, on world hunger, on human health, and on animals compiled from John Robbins's book, *The Food Revolution: How Your Diet Can Help Save Your Life and the World*—the most important and powerful book on food I have ever read. For the sake of this chapter, however, I'll share just a few:[9]

- Amount of water required to produce 1 pound of California foods, according to soil and water specialists at the University of California Agricultural Extension, working with livestock farm advisors:

1 pound of potatoes	24 gallons
1 pound of wheat	25 gallons
1 pound of chicken	815 gallons
1 pound of beef	5,214 gallons

- Number of calories of fossil fuel expended to produce 1 calorie of protein from soybeans: 2
- Number of calories of fossil fuel expended to produce 1 calorie of protein from beef: 54
- Number of people whose food energy needs can be met by the food produced on 2.5 acres of land:

If the land is producing rice	19 people
If the land is producing wheat	15 people
If the land is producing chicken	2 people
If the land is producing beef	1 person

In terms of crops, our monoculture farms survive because we spray them with massive quantities of pesticides and chemical fertilizers that not only poison the soil but also our waterways. Now we face a new, growing danger—genetic engineering. Whether or

---

8. Julia Whitty, "The Fate of The Ocean," *Mother Jones* (March/April 2006): 37.

9. While I have not included citations, each statistic is sourced and referenced in Robbins's book: *The Food Revolution: How Your Diet Can Help Save Your Life and The World* (San Francisco: Conari Press, 2002).

not genetically modified organisms (GMOs) are a significant threat to human health is debatable (though precaution is clearly in order), but we know that these plants are able to reproduce themselves, and we are unable to contain them. Those GMOs that have pesticides engineered into their genes will inevitably propel the evolution of super-resistant pests to which few—if any—crops will be immune since we have manufactured their diversity out of them. GMOs are currently contaminating organic crops, making it ever more difficult to ensure that at least some food is unadulterated.

The many problems caused by modern food production, articulated comprehensively and powerfully in Christopher Cook's *Diet for a Dead Planet*, are enormous, but fortunately there are groups committed to creating positive changes, and you will find not only further reading but also helpful websites in part III. Beyond learning more, however, what is a conscientious consumer to do? Small organic farmers have to compete with huge corporate agribusinesses but don't receive the subsidies that the corporations do, often making their foods expensive and out of reach for large numbers of people. The higher cost of organics leaves many people, especially those living in poor neighborhoods, with few or no supermarkets or food co-ops nearby, and few or no healthy choices in their small corner stores.

It may sound bizarre to suggest that U.S. citizens do not have enough choice in their diet given that in the United States and other affluent nations, supermarkets are practically the size of football fields, with row upon row of "choices." But the state of agribusiness and corporate consolidation actually limits choices insidiously. As Frances Moore Lappé writes in her book *Democracy's Edge*, "The choice most ... do *not* have is that of fresh, pesticide-free, whole foods at attractive prices in conveniently located stores."[10] Lappé includes the following sobering U.S. food facts and statistics as well:[11].

---

10. Frances Moore Lappé, *Democracy's Edge* (San Francisco: Jossey-Bass, 2006), 189.

11. While Lappé cites U.S. statistics, many countries face similar challenges and/or are influenced by the U.S. through trade policies. Some poor countries pay their debts in food production to wealthy countries while many in their population starve. Pesticide regulations are more lax in poor countries, though more protective in Western Europe.

- *Taxpayers subsidize the narrowing of choice.* Federal farm subsidies amount to an average of $19 billion every year—totaling $75 billion from 2000 to 2003. Their primary effect is to reduce costs for giant, food processing companies, not to help struggling family farmers. Since 1995, three-quarters of the funds have gone to the largest 10 percent of farms. Two-thirds of our family farmers get no subsidies at all.
- *Paying for illness.* Overall, one out of every eleven health dollars goes toward treating obesity-related conditions.
- *Pesticide harm.* Pesticides poison between ten and twenty thousand farm workers a year (and those are only the reported cases). The average American carries residues of at least thirteen pesticides, concludes a Centers for Disease Control study. One insecticide, Dursban (Dow Chemical), was found on average at levels three to five times above what the government deems "acceptable." In another study, preschoolers fed standard fare carried in their bodies six times the byproducts of dangerous pesticides—those implicated in mental and physical impairment—compared to children eating organic food.[12]

Again, this is where our voices come in. We can accept the problems listed above because it is true that, in the United States and many other wealthy countries, food is relatively cheap; and if you live in a middle class or affluent neighborhood, supermarkets are certainly well-stocked, even though they may be poorly stocked with affordable, ecological, organic whole foods. We can try to forget that pesticide-sprayed, genetically engineered, factory-farmed, processed, overpackaged food comes at an enormous expense to our health, animals, the environment, and farmers (and ultimately isn't cheap at all if we factor in the taxes we have to pay to clean up the ecological mess and provide health care to the hundreds of thousands succumbing to diet-related diseases every year). Or we can pressure our legislators to stop subsidizing corporate agribusiness and make polluters pay for the

---

12. Frances Moore Lappé, *Democracy's Edge* (San Francisco: Jossey-Bass, 2006), 198–199.

environmental cleanup costs associated with this form of farming. We can fight for real protections for animals. After all, what is done routinely to farmed animals in the United States would be illegal if done to a dog, cat, or parakeet. We can also join Community-Supported Agriculture (CSA) farms and food co-ops, as mentioned in earlier chapters, and put our dollars to work for change.

Periodically, we hear about a particular food and its effects. When migrant farm workers received media attention for picking table grapes under horrendous conditions, a boycott of these grapes ensued. When a hazardous chemical sprayed on apples was the subject of a *60 Minutes* program, public outcry followed, and many people boycotted apple juice until the chemical was banned. When the milk-fed veal industry gained notoriety for its cruel confinement of calves (as was previously described), many stopped eating veal. This boycott, along with citizen pressure, has created change. The European Union has banned veal crates, and Arizona has been the first state in the United States to outlaw them as well. But boycotts are only the beginning.

We also create change through "buycotts," that is, by buying healthy and humane foods. If pesticide-sprayed apples are dangerous, we can buy organic apples and apple juice. Our costs will be higher, but we can buy less and supplement our juice with the healthiest drink of all: water. If we learn that there is cruelty in the veal industry, we can consider new food choices that don't cause suffering.[13]

If you have a food co-op or a natural foods supermarket in your area but have avoided it because the costs are higher, try visiting again. While many of the costs will indeed be higher (because, as described above, small organic farmers are not subsidized with tax dollars the way huge agribusinesses are and cannot compete on volume), some items may be more afford-

---

13. It's important to mention, however, that substituting another animal food, such as chicken or turkey, for veal, actually contributes to greater animal suffering. Some people have told me that they'd never eat veal because of the cruelty in the industry, but eating chicken or turkey instead unwittingly creates more suffering, since poultry are such small animals that many more are produced and killed for every calf.

able than you thought, such as bulk organic grains, beans, cereals, and more. Another option is to visit farmers' markets, and join a local buying club or cooperative. In the club I joined, I received a monthly catalog that featured almost everything available at a large natural grocery (with the exception of fresh produce), and I ordered in bulk what I wanted for the month. Sometimes I split an order with another member if I didn't want so much of one item.

Ultimately, the solution to the problems of modern agriculture will come from a combination of the 3 *V*s (again, our **Voice**, our **Vote**, and our monetary **Veto**). By buying and eating healthier and more sustainably, ethically produced foods; and by asking your supermarket to stock these foods; and by pressuring elected officials to change laws and policies, we help change destructive and inhumane systems into ones that are healthy, compassionate, and ecologically friendly.

• • •

I grew up eating a fairly typical "American" diet of the 1960s and 1970s. Breakfast was usually some sugary cereal or glazed donuts with a glass of Tropicana orange juice. Lunch was whatever the cafeteria served up at school—creamed tuna, shepherd's pie, hot dogs and hamburgers, and cake or pie for dessert. Dinner was always some form of meat, starch, canned or frozen vegetables, and a salad, accompanied by a glass of milk that I was required to drink. Snacks and desserts included candy, Doritos, Sara Lee and Entenmann's cakes, sugary yogurt, soda, and ice cream. I never ate foods that had more than a few spices, whole grain bread or whole wheat pasta, and certainly no soy products.

In 1981 I decided not to eat mammals and birds anymore. I had always loved animals, and I was vaguely aware of the suffering they underwent in modern agriculture. When I realized that there was no significant difference between my dog (whom I would never eat) and a cow, pig, chicken, turkey, or sheep, I could not justify my food choices to myself anymore. I really didn't want to participate in causing pain, fear, and death to sentient beings if I did not have to. This choice did not present much of a culinary challenge, but nine years later, having learned about the suffering of dairy cows and their calf (veal) offspring, hens in the egg industry, and marine animals killed by the billions, I decided to stop eating dairy products, eggs, and sea animals to become a complete vegetarian (vegan). This necessitated overhauling my food choices. Soy, almond, and rice milk replaced cow's milk; a variety of ethnic dishes replaced typical American fare; whole grains replaced white flour and white rice; tofu and tempeh (a fermented soy food) became staples; fresh fruits and vegetables replaced canned and frozen foods; and my taste buds happily adjusted. Slowly but surely, I stopped enjoying highly processed foods and preferred whole foods; I stopped missing meat and cheese, and started craving the risottos or whole wheat pasta dishes I had learned to prepare. I came to love the sweetness of steamed kale.

I tell you these stories about myself with the hope that they will inspire you to question your assumptions about food. I have a friend who refuses to eat tofu. She is neither allergic nor sensitive to soy products, but she won't touch the stuff. No matter what I've prepared—banana cream pie, pasta sauce, onion dip for crackers, chocolate pudding—if it has tofu in it, she won't try it. I have accommodated her wishes (as so many people have accommodated my dietary choices over the many years I've been a complete vegetarian in a meat-eating culture), but it strikes me as silly to have such a closed attitude toward a particular food unless that attitude stems from deep conviction. If she had religious, ethical, or health concerns, I would feel entirely differently, but her attitude amounts, in my mind, to an irrational prejudice. She is not the first person I've met to react to tofu in this way, just like she's not the first to react to a new vegetable this way. In fact, she reminds me of myself as a child who did not want to try new foods. Foods create visceral responses. But if I can change from a TV dinner-eating, fast food-loving, sweet tooth-obsessed person with a twenty-year history of nonorganic, processed, high-salt, high-fat, high-sugar food into a whole food, organic, vegan junkie, well, anyone can—if they want to.

The question is, do you want to change your food choices to reflect your values? This may be the toughest question in this book because modifying what we eat can be very challenging, as everyone who has gone on a diet knows. When I decided to become vegan, saying goodbye to cheese pizza, bagels with cream cheese, and ice cream was not always easy. My values were sometimes in conflict with my desires. Fortunately, ingenuity, along with profit-driven companies who also have an ethic of social responsibility, has emerged to produce a plethora of meat and dairy alternatives that are delicious, organic, and nongenetically engineered. I now partake of Purely Decadent (a soy-based frozen dessert that I think tastes better than ice cream), soy cheese pizzas, and more. These, of course, aren't the healthiest of vegan options either, processed and packaged as they are, but they allow me to stay aligned with MOGO living when I'm too busy to prepare a meal or dessert from scratch. Now scientists are endeavoring to grow animal tissue in a lab, effectively producing meat without the animal. Perhaps this will turn out to be a MOGO solution, one that solves a host of problems associated with animal agriculture.

I began the previous paragraph asking whether you wanted to change your diet so that your food choices better reflect your emerging MOGO values. You may or may not; or you may sort of want to and sort of not want to; or you may want to, but may also want to eat your favorite foods. What I didn't yet discuss is how your answer to this question is not simply about the affect of your food choices on others. This book promised more than a path toward a peaceful world; it offered the promise of inner peace. So what do your food choices have to do with inner peace? Imagine four different people who regularly eat rice and beans:

- José eats rice and beans because that is what he's grown up eating his whole life. Rice and beans don't bring any special sort of inner peace; they're just dinner.
- Jack eats rice and beans because that is all he can afford. Rice and beans don't bring inner peace at all. In fact, they are a constant reminder of his financial hardships.

🍃 Jamala eats rice and beans because her doctor recommended them after she was diagnosed with a heart condition. Rice and beans don't bring much in the way of inner peace; they're more like medicine.

🍃 Jing, however, eats rice and beans because this diet is aligned with her values. Nourishing her body, mind, and spirit, Jing is full of joy and inner peace when she sits down to eat her meal.

In other words, your food choices, when you actively decide to align them with your values, help you cultivate inner peace; joy; satisfaction; and physical, mental, and spiritual health. If Jack, for example, came to view rice and beans as a reflection of his values rather than a symbol of his economic status, he might find greater satisfaction in his diet. If Jamala came to view rice and beans as healthy not only for her body but also for her soul, she might feel greater joy as she ate her meals. And if José recognized that his culture's staple foods contributed to healthy bodies and a healthy world, he might take great pride in modeling such positive choices.

I am not trying to suggest that my particular diet is the most likely to bring inner peace, or be the most sustainable, healthy, and humane for everyone. It represents my own effort to make food choices that do the most good and the least harm to myself, animals, the environment, and other people. You will need to determine your own MOGO diet. The challenge is not to let your taste buds, food fads, trends, advertising, and mainstream diets stand in the way of your willingness to learn and choose deliberately. If you decide to modify your food choices with the MOGO principle in mind, you may face some initial challenges, but if you try several different dishes, you are likely to find a few that you and everyone in your household enjoy.

If you begin to make MOGO food choices, you will likely discover some delightful personal benefits. You may come down with fewer colds and illnesses because your immune system will be supported by vitamins and minerals often absent in processed and fast food; and because your body will not be so stressed by excessive exposure to toxins, drug residues, hormones, and pesticides that become concentrated in animal flesh. You may also lose excess weight because you will probably be consuming fewer calories if you choose a healthier, more humane diet than is the norm in the United States and increasingly in other industrialized countries. Choosing foods with the goal of doing the most good and the least harm leads not only to peaceful eating but also to better health. What is best for others turns out to be best for us.

Practical Tips on Choosing Foods That Do the Most Good and the Least Harm

- Learn about your food. This is the most important step in making healthy, humane, and sustainable food choices. You'll find plenty of books, periodicals, films, and websites listed in part III that will help you learn what you need to know.
- As often as possible, choose foods that are:
  - Locally and organically produced
  - Produced through fair trade practices
  - Produced without cruelty to animals
  - Plant-based
  - Unprocessed
  - Not overly packaged, and if packaged, only in recycled and recyclable materials
  - Low in saturated fats and cholesterol
  - Produced without refined sugars and without hydrogenated vegetable oils
  - Made from whole grains
  - In season
- Make the choices above by joining a food co-op, cooperative buying club, or CSA; by shopping at natural foods supermarkets; and/or by visiting farmers' markets.
- Read labels, and learn what the ingredients are and what they imply in terms of their effects on animals, people, the environment, and you.

- Allow the criteria of kindness, compassion, and wisdom to enter into your food choices. Consider the world your food choices create.
- Try different kinds of foods. Most of us stick with tried and true dietary choices even if they aren't the most healthy, humane, or sustainable. Taste buds can joyfully change, however.

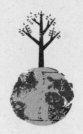

5. Work

Many of us know someone who gave up her high-powered, high-paying job to follow a dream of more fulfilling, meaningful work, and practically always the person is now happier and more joyful. Such people may face challenges and struggle with a lack of the security to which they have grown accustomed, but few want to return to what they have left behind. For example, consider Lynn Benander's story:

A year and a half ago, I quit my job to build a consumer-owned cooperative that would create community-owned energy resources. I saved up $12,000, kissed my paycheck goodbye, and set out on a journey. It was the best career move I ever made.

Since then I've been working with great colleagues, over 100 volunteers, a great board of directors, an awesome group of 250 members, and 3,000 dedicated supporters. Together we've developed a cooperative that both increases local access to existing clean-energy products and creates new sources. When people join Co-op Power, they tap into our network of contractors who install systems ranging from solar hot water to solar electric to wind to geothermal to small hydro. Low-income members can get volunteer installers and lower equipment costs to make these systems even more affordable.[1]

In addition to knowing people who've left unfulfilling jobs for purposeful work, I also know people who have decided *not* to pursue the vocation of their dreams specifically because they had the skills to earn a lot of money, and they wanted financial solvency for the primary purpose of donating to organizations working for social change. In fact two such people have crossed my path in recent years: One left a very compelling and personally interesting academic career to work in the lucrative tech industry and make substantial financial contributions to several nonprofit groups. Another was passionate about humane education but realized he was a better businessman than teacher, and could help the humane education field grow through his monetary donations to the field.

Then there are entrepreneurs who use their enormous creative talents for the good of others because doing so fulfills their desired epitaph. In their book, *The Power of Unreasonable People*, John Elkington and Pamela Hartigan quote David Green, a man they describe as a brilliant entrepreneur who brings modern health care technologies to the world's poorest people. David Green responded to a question about why he doesn't apply his great skills to making himself more money, saying, "My reasons are purely selfish. I figure I have been put on this earth for a very short period of time. I could apply my talents to making lots of money, but where would I be at the end of my lifetime? I would much rather be remembered for having made a significant contribution to improving the world into which I came than for having made millions."[2]

Not all of us have the ability to leave our job for something less secure; to simply choose to make loads of money; to be a brilliant, innovative entrepreneur; or to find work that is meaningful, pays a decent wage, and best utilizes our skills. Yet we can, to greater and lesser degrees, commit to what Buddhists call

---

1. Lynn Benander, quoted in "Community-Scale Energy," *Orion* (May/June 2007): 12.

2. John Elkington and Pamela Hartigan, *The Power of Unreasonable People* (Boston: Harvard Business School Press, 2008), 4.

"right livelihood." Right livelihood means pursuing work and careers that do no harm and that help others. In Jainism, an ancient religion that originated in India and which holds *Ahimsa* ("dynamic harmlessness") as one of its primary tenets, adherents are instructed to do work that is a force for good, and does not hurt other people, animals, or the environment.

Imagine a world in which people refused work that caused harm and suffering. Companies that were destructive or abusive to others would cease to exist. I am not so naïve as to rely on this approach as the sole initiative to stop polluting, habitat-destroying, and exploitive businesses, but thinking in terms of our own ability to make a difference through acting from our own integrity in relationship to our work is empowering and liberating.

A project called the "Graduation Pledge Alliance" is inspiring the next generation to make their work meaningful and helpful. Students at over one hundred colleges and universities have signed the pledge that reads: "I pledge to explore and take into account the social and environmental consequences of any job I consider, and will try to improve these aspects of any organizations for which I work." Pledge signers have turned down jobs, that are destructive and have made positive changes at other jobs, where they have brought the values of justice and sustainability to the companies where they work. I find such a movement of young people entering the workforce very exciting. Even if pledge signers are still few in number, the impact they make will not only directly influence company trends but will also inspire others.[3]

Big changes are necessary if we are to reverse the destruction that we are perpetuating, and such changes are the ones that are the most exhilarating and transformative. Given the hours most of us devote to work, what we choose to do through our careers and jobs may be the most significant way in which we can impact the world positively. We need companies, institutions, and governments to:

- Begin using wind, solar, geothermal, and/or other soon-to-be-developed renewable, nonpolluting energies

---

3. To find out more, visit http://www.graduationpledge.org.

- Take a leadership role on human rights, environmental preservation, and animal protection, and publicize their approaches so that these issues gain significant media attention that inspires other companies, organizations, and institutions to follow suit
- Create products that do not harm people, animals, or ecosystems, and which actively improve, protect, and restore the environment.
- Educate employees so they can become pioneers in humane and sustainable living
- Be on the forefront of green-collar jobs that not only repair the environmental damage we have caused but also create profitable work for a new generation of employees

Big as they may appear, these ideas are being implemented by people every day through their work and career choices. The following brief profiles provide a few examples.

Ray Anderson

When Ray Anderson, CEO of the carpet company Interface, learned about the negative environmental consequences of his company's manufacturing, he overhauled production to turn Interface into an environmental role model. He has been working not only to make his company less environmentally destructive but also to achieve an entirely nonpolluting business that will be a model for all manufacturers. Anderson has been called "the greenest chief executive in America," proving that with information, commitment, and care, we can transform businesses and manufacturing processes from ones that are destructive to ones that are sustainable and safe.

Jay Harman

Jay Harman, founder of PAX Scientific, an engineering research and development firm that specializes in finding innovative, streamlined solutions for industrial problems, has built a company whose purpose is to create sustainable products that reduce energy use in industrial systems.[4] Relying on the concept of bio-mimicry (that is, asking how nature would do it), PAX Scientific has created technologies that are dramatically more efficient and less energy intensive than those in mainstream use today.

Katie Redford

Katie Redford was a second-year law student when she went to Burma, and discovered the human rights abuses perpetrated by a military dictatorship securing a pipeline through Burmese villages for the California oil company Unocal. She wrote a paper in law school about the illegality of such actions and the need to sue, only to find her professor rejecting her arguments. Katie and her husband, Ka Hsaw Wa, a human rights activist who fled his native Burma, eventually brought a suit against Unocal. In 1997 the court concluded that corporations and their executive officers can be held legally responsible under the Alien Tort Claims Act for violations of international human rights norms in foreign countries, and that U.S. courts have the authority to adjudicate such claims. This was a landmark victory that set a crucial precedent for suing corporations for their human rights violations abroad.[5]

John Abrams

John Abrams started the South Mountain Company, a design and construction firm that creates eco-friendly buildings largely from salvaged wood and relies on environmental design.[6] John works on affordable housing projects, and has made his firm entirely employee-owned to guarantee that anyone who makes a career at South Mountain Company can share in the privileges, responsibilities, and rewards (as well as the headaches) of ownership. Letting go of sole ownership and control was challenging for John

---

4. See http://www.paxscientific.com.

5. See http://www.earthrights.org.

6. See http://www.somoco.com.

but has resulted in not only a better, more equitable company but also a commitment to promoting employee ownership globally.

Majora Carter

Majora Carter started Sustainable South Bronx, an organization dedicated to both restoring the blighted South Bronx (where Majora grew up) and to inspiring solutions in other impoverished city neighborhoods across the globe.[7] Majora connects the alleviation of poverty directly to the environment. Her organization creates solutions for our most persistent urban public health and global climate concerns, while providing skilled green-collar jobs for the largely disenfranchised people living in her community.

Paul Anastas

Paul Anastas got his Ph.D. in chemistry. Trained like most chemists, he was not taught to consider the effects of a chemistry career on our health or the environment. But Paul was inspired to create a new field called "Green Chemistry," a term he coined while working for the U.S. Environmental Protection Agency. Paul is now director of Yale University's Center for Green Chemistry and Green Engineering.

• • •

What do Ray Anderson, Jay Harman, Katie Redford, John Abrams, Majora Carter, and Paul Anastas have in common? They have all devoted their work and careers to making a positive difference. Whether you are a health care worker, lawyer, teacher, businessperson, or are involved in some other field, you can try to influence the course your company, school, firm, or institution takes. Many of us are in a position to make significant, positive choices through our work. The public relations executive does not have to accept the account from a fast food giant or tobacco

---

7. See http://www.ssbx.org.

company. There may be repercussions, and it is easy enough for such a person to say, "They'll just find another agency if we don't do it," yet someone who is in the exalted position to actually be an executive at a PR firm is also someone who has choices.

If you work for a company, organization, or institution that you cannot support ethically, what options are available to you? Often, we may feel like we have few choices because there are few jobs available in our region or we believe we will have to take a substantial pay cut to do good work. While this is sometimes true, you might surprise yourself. The world needs solutions to problems, and a growing population of people wants more humane choices. Jay Harman, Ray Anderson, Majora Carter, and John Abrams all demonstrate this. You, and all those who want to create a peaceful world, are in that market, hungry for options that let you put your money where your ethics are. Perhaps you might be one of the entrepreneurs creating successful businesses and products that serve this market. Many will succeed financially in their effort to create sustainable buildings, energy sources, forms of transportation, and agriculture, and do so by developing products that are ecologically friendly and humane. Even some of the biggest multinational corporations have CEOs who argue that more ethical, environmental, and peaceful choices will improve the bottom line.

We can also make choices at our existing workplaces that make a difference. If you work in an office, school, health care facility, or institution, what could you do to help your workplace make better choices? For instance, how might your office reduce paper consumption? Could you help find recycled paper, and set up a recycling system so that office paper does not wind up in a landfill or incinerator? If your office provides coffee for employees, could you influence the brand that is purchased so that you are drinking fair trade, organic, shade-grown coffee?[8] What about energy consumption? Could your office lower the thermostat in

---

8. I've already discussed the concepts of fair trade and organic. "Shade grown" refers to coffee grown *within* rainforests rather than on plantations where rainforests were cleared for agriculture. Coffee plants naturally grow under rainforest canopies.

127

the winter and raise it in the summer to conserve fuel? Could you install compact fluorescent light bulbs? Could you suggest different cleaning products in the bathroom—ones that are not tested on animals and that are nontoxic? Or different toilet paper, from companies that use 100 percent recycled paper?

For some of us, these simple suggestions are off-putting. We may not want to be perceived as the activist in the office or carry the responsibility for changes, especially if we perceive them to be too small to be significant. Yet it can feel great to set healthy standards and to have an office model positive change. When people help their offices implement these kinds of changes, they usually find it very rewarding and satisfying. And as long as they present their ideas in a positive, helpful manner, they are generally well received by their supervisors. Most companies and institutions are glad to be trailblazers as long as the costs are not prohibitive, and especially if the choices are cost-effective or even profitable. It is not as if executives want to pollute, hurt other people, destroy forests, or harm animals. And usually, those in charge of supplies, custodial care, purchasing, and so on, are simply unaware of the better choices that may be available. Whether through a big career change or small, daily choices where you work, you can make a difference that creates more peace of mind for you through your work and a better world for all.

Practical Tips for Work That Does the Most Good and the Least Harm

Take time to identify your values:

- 🍃 Take stock of your job or career. Is your work doing more than paying the bills? Is it work that is fulfilling? Does it align with your values? Does it best utilize your skills? If you decide that you do not want to stay in your job, practice the 3 *I*s regarding your future work life. **Inquire** about options. What resources are available to you to launch a new career or business? What good and realistic ideas and possibilities do you have? **Introspect** and determine where your skills and passions meet, considering those risks you are willing to take. Choose to live with **integrity** in relation to your work choices.

- If you want to stay in your present job, consider what you might do (as described above) to improve the ways in which your company or institution operates, and the products or services it produces. Make sure to communicate your ideas with clarity, respect, helpfulness, and openness.
- Volunteer where you would like to work. Many institutions hire from within, and if you show initiative and talent, and have demonstrated hard work and commitment, you may be the next person hired.

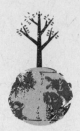

6. Activism, Volunteerism, and Democracy

Throughout the book I have asked you to evaluate (and where appropriate, modify) your lifestyle, work, purchases, diet, and daily decisions. While I've periodically stated that personal choice-making will not by itself easily or efficiently change systems that are oppressive and destructive, I have nonetheless urged you to make choices with as much integrity as you can. If we do not personally model the message we hope to convey to the greatest possible extent, and if we don't put our money and our work time where our ethics lie, corporations and governments are unlikely to lead in these efforts on their own. Yet, as **Key 4—Model Your Message and Work for Change** describes, we need to do more. To create positive, systemic change quickly and effectively, we must take action, volunteer our time, and participate in the democratic process.

For many of us, the image of an activist is an angry, sign-toting, slogan-chanting protester. Those are the activists the media often portrays. But there are many different ways to be an activist—that is, someone active on behalf of others, a change-maker. If the opposite of an activist is one who is passive, then all who endeavor to create a better world, rather than passively accepting the status quo, are activists.

When I realized that I was not inclined to be a traditional activist (the protest-attending sort who stood on street corners with signs), I initially thought poorly of myself. Surely I could muster the effort to be an activist on behalf of issues I cared about, even if I disliked the actual activities. Protests and marches are often very effective and important ingredients in the mix for creating change. Imagine if Martin Luther King Jr. had not given his "I have a dream speech" at the 1963 civil rights march in Washington, D.C. But I suspect that there are readers of this book who believe, as I did, that protesting and marching define activism, and who feel that such activities are not for them. It would be tragic if such people failed to recognize the many opportunities they have to contribute to positive change.

When I expanded my own definition of activism, and discovered a way to mix my passions and talents in service to a greater good, I was able to give more than I'd imagined. Although I still sometimes attend marches and protests, I have found ways to create change that are better suited to my personality, use more of my skills, allow me to contribute more effectively, and have a greater positive impact.

Each of us can assess our talents and passions, and find the place where they meet. The following questions will help you. It is important to actually write down your answers,[1] because to implement them you will need to give these questions your thoughtful attention rather than a cursory glance. These are questions that can help you direct your life toward choices that are not only deeply fulfilling to you but which will make a difference for others.

1. What issues or problems most concern you? Are you particularly drawn to solve problems such as poverty, inadequate

---

1. You may wish to begin a MOGO journal in which you not only answer these questions (as well as complete the **MOGO Questionnaire and Action Plan** in part III) but which you also use to implement the 3 *I*s. This journal can be a place to write down information you acquire through your inquiry, to put into words the thoughts that arise when you introspect, and to explore the ways in which you can then put this information and your self-awareness into action to further your integrity.

education, child abuse, food insecurity, genetic engineering, animal cruelty, global climate change, sweatshop labor, escalating worldwide slavery, peak oil, media monopolies, HIV/AIDS, nuclear weapons, genocide, resource depletion, pollution? Is there a community issue that you feel passionately about? Beyond your family and friends, who and what do you care most about?

2. What skills and talents do you have that could be combined with your concerns above to enable you to make a difference?
3. What specific steps could you take to bring your talents and concerns together to achieve your goals?
4. If you are already an activist or changemaker, are you best using your time and talents to make sure that you are as effective as you can be? What might you be doing that would better utilize your skills and maximize your impact?

As you answered these questions, did you find a specific issue beckoning you, or did you realize that you are concerned about many issues most of which intersect and interrelate? Some of us are drawn to a single issue. Others care broadly about many issues but none so strongly that they compel us to action. But if we realize that we have talents and experiences that we can bring to bear, and if we then witness the good that can come when our skills are appropriately focused, we also discover the joy that comes in solving entrenched problems.

Imagine how much might change if every person took the time to reflect upon the issues that deeply concern them and then examine the skills they have to bring about positive change. Many more coalitions would form among people who care about the same issues, but who could offer a range of talents and experiences. More skilled professionals wanting to bring their knowledge forward to solve problems would identify ways they could make a substantial difference.

For example, let's imagine a successful marketer reads this book and writes down her concerns. She has two children, and she is worried about their education. In her opinion, the emphasis on standardized tests is squelching their creativity and love of learning. The local school has cut its arts and music program to focus more attention on passing mandatory, multiple-choice tests, and her children are now miserable at school.

This mom decides to do something about her concerns. She joins the PTA, talks to teachers and school administrators, and reaches out to other parents to hear their perspectives. She discovers that most share her concerns.

Next, she writes down her skills. Because of her marketing background, she knows how to influence ideas. She realizes that she will have to address her concerns at the national level (where federal laws that impact her children's education are made) and contact her senators and representatives, but in the meantime she decides to use her knowledge and talents to try to restore the arts and music program at her children's school. By meeting with all the stakeholders, focusing their concerns into a few clear phrases, engaging the school board, and using her contacts to present the issue in a creative manner in the local media, this mother influences the school board to revitalize the art and music programs. Her success then fuels further involvement beyond her local community to help improve schools and education for all children.

If my imaginary scenario above seems unrealistic to you, then consider this real-life account: Henry Spira, who worked alone, without a big organization or staff, significantly changed the course of product testing on animals. In 1980 he took out a full-page ad in *The New York Times* that read, "How many rabbits does Revlon blind for beauty's sake?" The accompanying photo of a blinded rabbit caught people's attention and sparked a remarkably rapid change in product testing. While many of the big companies producing personal care and cleaning products do continue to test their products on animals, Revlon and many others stopped such tests in favor of nonanimal alternatives, and hundreds of small companies began producing personal care products without ever doing animal tests.[2] Henry's success garnered donations to further his

---

2. For a list of companies that do and do not test their products on animals, visit http://www.caringconsumer.com/resources_companies.asp.

efforts, but he continued to work primarily on his own, successfully changing the policies of large, multinational corporations and influencing new companies.[3]

I recently watched the PBS series *The New Heroes*,[4] which documents fourteen individuals who have made a stunning difference for others and the environment. These inspired and committed individuals have each combined their compassion with their skills to solve pervasive problems. Here are two examples:

Mohammad Yunus

Mohammad Yunus was an economics professor in the 1970s in Chitagong, Bangladesh, during his country's terrible famine. He would walk out the university doors and see people dying of starvation around him. He wondered what good all his knowledge of economics was if it was not helping these people. So Yunus visited a nearby village and asked the villagers what they needed. After a discussion, forty-two people told him they needed a combined $27 to start small businesses to prepare rice for market. He loaned them this money despite the fact that they had no collateral, and thus began a microcredit movement that has lifted millions of people out of poverty.

Yunus approached banks to ask why they didn't make such loans, and the answer was always the same: banks do not loan money to people without collateral. Yunus saw this principle—the more you have the more you get, and the less you have the less you get—as backwards. He started Grameen Bank, loaning small amounts of money to people with no collateral and offering

---

3. Many years ago, a close friend of mine launched what has since become an extremely successful company that produces personal care products. When she started the company, I asked her if she was going to conduct product tests on animals. She assured me she wasn't but not because she personally cared about this issue. She said that it simply wasn't wise from a business standpoint to participate in animal testing in today's climate. Consumers and citizen activists had changed business practices through their dollars and their voices.

4. Visit http://www.pbs.org/opb/thenewheroes/ to learn more or order a DVD of this inspiring series.

them convenient loan repayment plans. Yunus has lent billions of dollars to millions of people, mostly women who are poor and would otherwise not qualify for loans. Grameen's repayment rates are over 95 percent, and his model has been replicated around the world. Yunus, who once said that he wanted to be a stick in the wheels that would finally stop the infernal machine that keeps people in poverty, has since won the Nobel Peace Prize.

Albina Ruiz

Albina Ruiz runs the organization Healthy Cities in Peru. Horrified by her country's lack of waste treatment and the consequent suffering of its people, Ruiz sought to solve an entrenched, deadly problem. Poverty-stricken people in Peru have been living in and around garbage dumps, trying to eke out a meager living from the trash of others despite the dangerous, unhealthy, and unsanitary conditions. Still others across the country have faced the persistent problems that arise when 75 percent of trash is not disposed of properly. Ruiz wanted to create a win-win situation for Peruvians, and she continues to work hard to do so.

For those living in and around garbage dumps, Ruiz's organization is creating stable jobs for separating, utilizing, and treating recyclable items, organic waste, and trash. Now many people, once sickened by the garbage dumps, have good jobs with benefits as they simultaneously solve a national crisis. By creating other jobs in trash collection, Healthy Cities is not only increasing economic opportunities but also protecting those living downstream from cities that have traditionally dumped all their wastes into the river.[5]

• • •

These are just two profiles from the series *The New Heroes*. The series is not only an inspiration but also a reminder that each of

---

5. Visit http://www.pbs.org/opb/thenewheroes/ to learn more about this hero and others in the PBS series *The New Heroes*.

us can make a difference, too. These changemakers also provide examples of how activism can turn into meaningful work. There *is* money to be made in doing work that does good.

If the thought of starting an organization and taking on such big projects yourself sounds daunting, you can volunteer at existing groups that do work you believe in. Volunteerism is activism. You do not have to start your own organization, or develop your own campaign or movement to make a difference. Instead, you can plug into agencies that are eager for help from people like you.[6] There are international service organizations with branches all over the world. For example, Rotary International (rotary.org) is dedicated to helping improve the world through a range of service activities (including efforts to help those in Central America who are living in and around garbage dumps). With over one million members and with clubs in most cities, joining Rotary or another service group enables you to participate with community members on efforts that inspire you.

I've already touched on some forms of volunteerism in this book because volunteering helps build community, which is MOGO for you and others. We need volunteers not only to help existing institutions function at their best and provide the services people rely on, but also to help organizations and nonprofit groups envision and enact situational and systemic change. As I discussed in **Key 6—Take Responsibility**, we as individuals are often constrained by situations and systems that impair the possibilities of finding MOGO solutions. Volunteering for those groups that attempt to improve situations and modify systems so that they are more conducive to MOGO living and a MOGO future helps to bring about the kinds of changes that will enable more of us to actually lead MOGO lives.

One of the most important ways in which we can be active in positive change is by educating others. This is the form of changemaking I choose, and I believe that it's the foundation for all lasting change. When we teach, we give people the opportunity to grow intellectually and to make informed choices in their own lives.

---

6. Again, visit http://www.volunteermatch.org.

Teaching happens in obvious places like schools, universities, and religious institutions; through the media; and at adult learning centers, but it's taking place in other venues, too. Health care practitioners, counselors, artists, parents, friends, and involved, vocal citizens educate others all the time. Education is one of the easiest and most significant ways to start making a difference. Since you are always learning and teaching anyway, you might do so more deliberately by:

- Writing letters to the editor of newspapers and magazines, both print and online
- Posting a blog on your social networking site
- Starting a school club if you are a student and inviting speakers to present on various issues, as well as teaching what you know to your fellow students
- Hosting a film and discussion series in your home on human rights issues, food security, environmental preservation, animal protection, humane and sustainable living, and so on. Such films will introduce friends and neighbors to ideas for peaceful living that are not yet part of daily culture. (See the list of suggested videos in chapter 12, **Recommended Resources**.)
- Requesting opportunities to speak at local schools, places of worship, camps, service clubs, learning centers, senior centers, and so on. with a presentation on living a compassionate, peaceful life and creating a sustainable, humane world. If you are shy about speaking yourself, you can take the initiative, and invite experts to come and speak to such groups instead.
- Sharing books, pamphlets, videos, and websites with others who might benefit from learning some of what you have learned
- Starting or joining reading clubs, salons, and conversation cafés to learn from and share with others
- Taking on a cable access television program, and sharing your views and knowledge with a wide audience. One of the graduates of our M.Ed. program has hosted a cable access

show with his wife for many years.[7] Their excellent shows influence thousands of people.

🍃 Developing an email or phone tree in your community to keep people up to date on pending legislation or issues of concern in which they can take part

In addition to activism and volunteerism, we all need to become politically involved as participating members of democracies. David Orr, the professor mentioned in **Key 3—Make Connections and Self-Reflect** who asks his students about the connection between obesity and the dead zone in the Gulf of Mexico, puts the global challenges we face this way:

> Looking to the horizon, the political, social, and economic topography grows steeper and more treacherous. We will soon see the mounting consequences of climate change, the loss of biological diversity, toxic pollution, the breakdown of entire ecosystems, rising population, growing poverty, terrorism, ecological refugees, political instability, and new diseases for which we have no good remedies. . . . We now have to move quickly from fossil fuels to renewable energy and forestry, rebuild habitable cities, construct an ecologically viable transportation system, protect biological diversity, create sustainable communities, safeguard air and water quality, eliminate toxins, and not least, distribute wealth fairly within and between generations.[8]

After reading something as sobering as this, it's clear that choosing a toothbrush with a replaceable head, ensuring that your office recycles, or volunteering at your local environmental group—important though these kinds of activities are—must also be accompanied by political involvement for effective, meaningful, and timely *policy* changes.

---

7. See Neil and Annie Hornish's *Animal Matters* on Connecticut cable television.

8. David Orr, *The Last Refuge* (Washington, D.C.: Island Press, 2005), 5.

We must pressure our existing lawmakers and elect new ones to lead us toward a better future. This is the nature of democracy. Regardless of our political affiliation (or lack thereof), we must hold elected officials to the standard of visionary leadership that does not give in to special interests or bow to the pressures of the largest corporate contributor.

Ironically, there are those who call environmental protection a special interest, but consider paper and mining companies and corporate agribusiness representative of the mainstream value of economic growth. Industry lobbyists are well paid and plentiful, and real campaign finance reform has yet to happen in the United States. This means that we citizens have much work to do. If we shirk our democratic duties, we lose our voice and our capacity to influence policy changes.

Never before in my adult life has democracy been more actively practiced around the world. The internet has dramatically changed our ability to connect and has engaged millions of people. Youth are finally beginning to vote in the United States in greater numbers after decades of voting attrition. We have passed clean election laws in a few states, including my own state of Maine, enabling candidates without high personal incomes to run in elections while preventing them from being beholden to industry dollars. The internet is also providing sources of information to the public that have been kept out of mainstream media, so that at the same time as media consolidation is limiting our range of information on television, radio, and in newspapers, an open source of knowledge is ever more available from our homes, libraries, schools, and offices.

People sometimes doubt that their one voice matters very much, yet legislators will form a committee to examine an issue after receiving as few as ten letters on a subject. If you found ten friends willing to commit to sending their lawmakers a letter or email about an issue of mutual concern, you would have generated those ten letters (plus your own).

Frances Moore Lappé's *Democracy's Edge*, mentioned in chapter 4, is a hopeful, engaging, and compelling book that charts the multitude of ways in which people are practicing democracy and creating change. Reading this book, it is easy to find your own niche in participating in the democratic process.

Another important resource for those eager to engage politically is the New America Foundation (newamerica.org). This foundation outlines thoughtful policies for the United States in the twenty-first century. It is refreshing to read suggestions that are not aligned with a political party but are simply meant to offer solutions to specific challenges of our time—from public education and social security, to taxes and health insurance, to the democratic process itself. While I don't agree with all of their suggestions, this website offers visionary and practical perspectives to solve a host of problems. Both *Democracy's Edge* and the New America Foundation focus on political change in the United States, but the policies and ideas they explore can be used and expanded upon anywhere.

It is easy to feel disenfranchised from politics. Between the rhetoric, the dissembling, the corruption, and the outright lies, it can be hard to cast our votes, especially in national elections, without some sense of cynicism. But without our voices demanding accountability, honesty, and commitment to the future, we will not succeed in creating real change.

Many of our political leaders expect us to be selfish. They assume we will protest increases in fuel prices and decry rises in food costs, and therefore make sure that oil companies and huge agribusinesses are subsidized (presuming we won't notice that these subsidies come out of our wallets though taxes). Thinking ahead would mean that small, organic farmers and companies working on renewable energy sources might instead be the recipients of government investment.

Politicians generally expect that we would rather have endless conveniences than follow the precautionary principle[9] (to keep potentially hazardous chemicals out of our air, aquifers, soil, and

---

9. From http://www.en.wikipedia.org/wiki/Precautionary_principle: "The precautionary principle is a moral and political principle which states that if an action or policy might cause severe or irreversible harm to the public, in the absence of a scientific consensus that harm would not ensue, the burden of proof falls on those who would advocate taking the action."

products), and so they bow to the pressures exerted by large multinational chemical and oil companies. Buying trends, which are largely and falsely created through advertising and manipulation, lead us to believe that we would prefer more tax-subsidized chain stores, filled with the work of sweatshop laborers, to the more expensive—but better and humanely made—products available in our downtowns and through mail order companies. Many corporations prey on our insecurities and desire for love, happiness, and peace, associating their products with our wish for joy, and then politicians reinforce our manufactured desires by refusing to challenge these corporations' hegemony.

But I'm guessing that most readers of this book would prefer policies that protect people, the environment, animals, and a viable future for generations to follow. Millions of people share such values and commitments to a sustainable and safe future. If more of us were to let our elected officials know what we truly care about (and elect officials who truly represent us), policies would shift. "Big-box" stores would have to pay for the extra infrastructure, pollution cleanup, and other problems associated with their companies, and ensure that those who produce the products they sell are not exploited to keep costs to shoppers unreasonably and unsustainably low.

Companies would not be able to sell their growth hormones to dairy farmers (as one example) with such lax government oversight (or none at all), or keep the public from knowing which products do and do not contain these hormones. Nor would they be able to sue organic farmers whose fields become contaminated with genetically modified seeds through no fault of their own.[10]

The sooner we commit to a safe and sustainable future for everyone, and participate in democracy with this principle in mind, the sooner we will have the leadership to create policies that bring us closer to this goal. When long-term thinking, wisdom, compassion, honesty, and courage become the norm among

---

10. For more information about Monsanto's lawsuits against farmers whose fields are contaminated with Monsanto's patented seeds, visit http://www.percyschmeiser.com and watch the film, *The Future of Food* (Lily Films, 2004).

political leaders, and when special interests have no power over legislative and executive decision making, we will discover that it is possible to advance laws and policies that truly do the most good and the least harm.

Practical Tips on Becoming Active for Change

- After completing the questions at the beginning of this chapter, identify three to five ways in which you can bring your talents to bear on your concerns. Narrow these down to one that strikes you as likely to have the most positive impact. Then take action and do it. Later, choose another one on your list to take on.

- When you listen to, watch, or read the news and learn about a problem that concerns you, ask yourself: "What could I do about this?" Think of something practical and easy enough that you will do it. Be creative. Share the thought with ten friends.

- Ask your friends and colleagues about what they are involved in that they may never have told you about before. If an issue sparks your interest, join them in their efforts.

- Raise a concern at the dinner table with your family, at a pot-luck with your friends, around the cafeteria in your school or senior center, and/or at your suppers in your religious institution, and brainstorm ideas for what you could do to help. Make a group commitment.

- Put your current skills to use. A web designer could help an emerging nonprofit group create a website; a scientist could review data and offer accurate analysis and expertise; a teacher could incorporate all the issues in this book into the curriculum. Assess your talents and find your niche.

- If you're skilled at making money, donate to organizations and individuals with limited budgets that are working to create the changes that are most meaningful to you. Make sure to carefully evaluate the groups and people to whom you donate to ensure that they are using your money wisely and effectively.

- ✐ If you are a parent, join the PTA and get involved in your child's school. Work to bring humane education into the classroom (visit HumaneEducation.org).
- ✐ If you are a student, bring the issues in this book to your school by starting a MOGO club (visit HumaneEducation.org).
- ✐ If you're a senior citizen, bring the issues in this book to your community centers.
- ✐ Join a service club in your community, meet your neighbors, and get involved in global and local efforts to create positive change.
- ✐ Visit accuratedemocracy.com to learn more about the process and language of democracy. Then visit fairvote.org and learn about the Instant Runoff Voting (IRV) solution to the problem of rule by extreme factions.
- ✐ Volunteer for a candidate whose values and integrity reflect your own, or run for office yourself.
- ✐ Start calling, emailing, and writing to your elected officials to express your opinion about both specific legislation and general concerns. If you live in the United States, visit congress.org to contact your legislators and learn about their voting records.

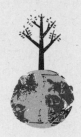

7. 10 Principles for a MOGO Life

This book has covered a lot of ground in a narrative format. So here is your condensed version for a quick way to think about choices that do the most good and the least harm (MOGO). Much of this list has been covered in the previous chapters; some information is new. Use it as a general guide and easy reference.

1. **Commit to the 3 *I*s: Inquire, Introspect, live with Integrity.** Expose yourself to information and ideas about MOGO living by talking to and learning from people from all walks of life—especially people who are also trying to do the most good and the least harm; by reading widely and deeply; by visiting websites aimed at making a difference; and by viewing relevant films. You can find a list of regularly updated websites, books, magazines, and films in the resources section at HumaneEducation.org. Then introspect: identify your values, consider what is most important to you, assess your talents and interests, and seek out ways to put these together practically and productively. Finally, live with integrity. To the best of your ability, put your values into practice.

2. **Work for change.** Give some of your time, resources, and talents to create systemic change that benefits all. Choose the

issues that most concern and compel you, get involved, and relish the joy that such generosity brings to yourself and others. If you can, make your career one that is MOGO.

3. **Rethink, Reuse, Repair, and Recycle.** As much as possible, rethink your use of products that are unnecessary, inhumane, produced through exploitive business practices, nonrecyclable, overpackaged, toxic, and/or unsustainable. When you do make purchases, choose the most sustainable, efficient, humane, fairly traded, and healthy versions. Then reuse what you can, repair what is reparable, and recycle when you are through. And in the midst of these 4 *R*s, consider what you could borrow instead of buy, and what you could share with friends and neighbors so that they can better rethink unnecessary products, too.

4. **Eat for life.** As much as possible, choose plant-based foods produced close to where you live, grown organically, and unprocessed. This will improve your health, the environment, the lives of animals, and the well-being of other people.

5. **Reduce your ecological footprint.** Drive less, carpool, walk, bike, car-share, and use public transportation more. If you need to own a car, choose one with the best fuel efficiency to meet your needs. Choose the most energy efficient and ecologically friendly options for homes, home repair, appliances, lighting, heating, and cooling. Choose your recreation and vacations with MOGO in mind as well: an ecotourism excursion over a cruise; cross-country skiing instead of downhill skiing; canoeing more often than motorboating.

6. **Transform education.** People need relevant information, tools for critical thinking, and motivation to lead meaningful lives that contribute to a better world. Whether you are a parent, student, teacher, elder, or concerned citizen, help make living sustainably and peacefully the very purpose of education at all levels by engaging in dialogue with lawmakers, educators, and school and university administrators.

7. **Invest your money ethically.** If you are going to rely on a mutual fund for retirement or college, choose a socially responsible investment fund. Ask for a portfolio and assess

whether the company invests in the kinds of businesses you want to support. Seek out community banks and credit unions, and consider microlending and investment in social businesses as a means of using your money to help others.

8. **Build community.** Find others who share your desire to make MOGO choices by joining existing groups or creating your own group, and invite people to join you. You will enjoy the friendship and camaraderie, and help make a difference at the same time. Don't forget the communities of which you are already a part. Get to know your neighbors, and work with them to make your neighborhood healthy, supportive, and safe.

9. **Teach others.** Share what you know with others and engage them in the challenge of living a MOGO life by using positive communication that does not judge or blame. Listen as often as you speak. Teaching and learning happen everywhere: one on one, in schools, in religious congregations, at camps, in families, in print and film, at learning centers, on social networking internet sites, at senior facilities, and so on. Model your message, and speak your truth in kind and inspiring ways wherever you are and with whomever you're in contact.

10. **Strive for balance.** Set reasonable goals for yourself, and remember that the "most good, least harm" equation includes you. You are a role model for a MOGO life, so find the balance that lets you live joyfully, enthusiastically, and compassionately.

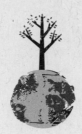

8. MOGO Stories

Now that you have arrived at the end of part II, I hope that you are enthusiastic and inspired to make MOGO the guiding principle in your daily choices, your work, and through engaged citizenship. Just as I ended part I with stories about individuals striving to find balance, I'm ending this section with stories from people who have attended our MOGO workshop, and who actively strive to lead MOGO lives. As you embark on the MOGO journey yourself, it's my hope that their voices will nourish, encourage, and inspire you.

MOGO has changed every aspect of my life. I now carefully consider major decisions like where to live (trying to find work closer to home or home closer to work); what kind of groceries to buy (organic versus conventional); who to buy them from (local CSA and farmers' market versus grocery store); how far things have had to be shipped to get to me; the conditions under which people have had to work to supply me with my needs and wants, and so on.

I also think much more about smaller decisions every day, like whether to take that extra two minutes at the grocery store to fill out an employee compliment form, to count to ten before fussing at the dog for eating my lunch (that I left unguarded on the counter for two seconds), to staying after church or a piano lesson to listen to someone in need of a friend.

Living according to the MOGO principle has made me more aware that every decision we make every day, no matter how seemingly insignificant, adds one more drop to the well of our lives. Every time I make a decision to help rather than hurt, my life is expanded and made more joyful. I have found clarity about what is truly important, and therefore have freed up an enormous amount of time and energy to use to better purposes. I have become aware of how often in the past I did not have the information I needed to consider how others' lives were affected by my every decision. I am grateful to realize that my desires do not entitle me to add to another's suffering. As a result, my desires have aligned more closely with my hopes for a better world.

—Lynne Westmoreland, New York

Writing my epitaph made me realize that if I want to achieve certain goals and live my values, now is the time. It was scary to think that I could die without having lived my epitaph. Now that I'm living my epitaph, I have much greater self-respect, inner peace, and a strong sense of integrity.

I've been actively cultivating a MOGO community. I joined a local cabaret theater in which we create skits, songs, and plays. I write and perform pieces about issues that are important to me, educating others while entertaining them, and have built a vibrant community of active and engaged friends at the same time.

Because the MOGO principle asks us to take responsibility while striving for balance, I feel encouraged to do the best I can without castigating myself for minor failures. I try to make the best choices based on what I currently know, and I strive to learn more so that I have more knowledge upon which to act.

—Amy Morley, Maine

The MOGO principle has helped me define my values and hone in on what types of actions best suit me. I'm better able to express my opinions while being sensitive to the needs of others. I now regularly communicate about challenges that concern me, and I work on legislative issues. I'm much more confident sharing my views and passing on information to colleagues, and have been encouraging my coworkers to take action on the issues that concern them, too. I've initiated a couple of environmental actions at my workplace (river cleanups, global warming events) and am challenging myself to take on more leadership roles. Plus, I'm more self-reflective and have a great sense of community now.

—**Monica Keady, Connecticut**

One of the biggest take-aways from MOGO is the realization that it is okay to acknowledge that I can't do it all, and that little steps really do make a difference. I used to feel that no matter what I did, it was never enough. If ever I do begin to feel restless in this area, I consider what I can add to my efforts, but now without guilt.

I've come to realize that my consumer choices have a huge impact in the world. Now I am very conscientious about where items that I purchase come from. I also have become more aware of which companies I want to support. I try to buy locally, reduce the amount of waste that I produce, reuse items whenever possible, and purchase used items instead of new items.

Finally, I look for opportunities to offer a kind word. Life is short, and I love saying something positive to someone.

—**Lisa Kaim, New Hampshire**

It can be easy for someone working for change to vilify other people who contribute to the *status quo* by way of their choices. It can be even easier to beat oneself up for going back to old habits now and then—perhaps due to lack of a better choice in a given situation, or perhaps just being tired from fighting existing systems constantly. Thus, for an agent of change, the MOGO principle is a welcome break that allows us to be kind and understanding to ourselves and others. In my life, the MOGO principle allows me to be at peace while working to make a positive difference. It provides a framework that allows me not only to self-reflect and set goals, but to connect with others and create change that benefits all.

—Kumara Siddhartha, MD, Massachusetts

• • •

It is not only adults whose lives change, improve, and become more meaningful when they adopt the MOGO principle. Recently, I taught a week-long MOGO class to a sixth- and seventh-grade class. We spent five mornings analyzing products, advertisements, and either/or thinking, and I invited the students to embrace the MOGO principle in relation to themselves, other people, animals, and the environment.

When I carried in my Aeropostale shopping bag of props on the first day, one of the girls shouted out, "I *love* Aeropostale! It's my favorite store!" I smiled. She didn't yet know that we'd be talking about how such brand loyalty develops, nor that the bag wasn't simply a container for other props but a prop itself. By the end of the week, after analyzing company messages, this same girl wrote the following on her personal MOGO plan, a questionnaire that allowed each student to consider how and in what ways they'd like to choose differently after a week of humane education:

- If I see an ad for something I like, I'll try to analyze it.
- Do some research on any products or stores I'm going to buy from.
- Start a club with kids my age to help everything go MOGO.
- Write letters every month on a cruel happening that shouldn't be happening.
- Make it known to other people what cruelty is going on and [tell them] how to stop it.
- Try not to watch as much television.

🖐 Help out at [the local food pantry] or any other charity I come to find needs my help.

Another girl in the class wrote that she's going to volunteer, shop less and recycle more, donate to her local shelter, and "work toward an equal rights world." One boy, who often seemed less engaged than other students and somewhat reluctant to do the assignments, surprised me on the last day. I had thought that he was simply tolerating the class, but when we were each sharing one thing from our MOGO plan, he said he was going to eat less meat, a subject we hadn't covered in any detail. I realized that he'd been far more engaged and concerned than I'd thought.

But as great as all their commitments were, perhaps the most exciting moment came when I asked the students a question about my book *Claude and Medea*, which they had read in class prior to my arrival. The novel revolves around the adventures of its seventh-grade protagonists who (illegally) rescue stolen dogs from a laboratory. I wanted to know if they thought what Claude and Medea had done was right or wrong. I felt like doing a jig when the first hand went up, and the boy who raised it said that he thought they were wrong to break the law, even for a good cause. I had told the kids at the beginning of the week not to believe me but to think for themselves. I had stressed that all opinions were welcome, even if they thought they were the only ones who held such an opinion.

It was clear that the students respected my opinion and wanted to learn what I had to teach, so it would not have been surprising had they suppressed their perspectives in favor of mine and the majority. But instead I saw a class full of respectful critical thinkers, eager to listen and learn, but equally committed to their own capacity to make MOGO decisions based on their own beliefs and values. These students fully embraced the 3 *I*s, brought their own inquiry to the subjects we covered, introspected without fear of reprisal for difference, and spoke their truth with integrity. Nothing could have made me happier as a humane educator. Such young people are the greatest hope for a better future.

Two months later, I taught a week-long MOGO class to the eighth grade at this same school. While we discussed such problems as poverty, human slavery, environmental degradation, and animal cruelty, we spent most of our time learning about people like Mohammad Yunus and Albina Ruiz (mentioned in chapter 6, **Activism, Volunteerism, and Democracy**), who are changing systems and solving problems, and we discussed what each of us could do to be part of positive change, too. These students also completed a MOGO plan and sent me letters after the class was over. Here's what some wrote:

> Spending that week with you was the most inspiring five days of my life so far. You made me realize how much just one person can do to help the world and how much more you can do by educating others about the issues. I have already started teaching my parents about how to make MOGO choices. It really feels good to know that I can take sometimes simple and sometimes complex actions to save a life and our world. Thank you so much for this opportunity! I will carry that week with me for a lifetime.

• • •

> Thank you so much for coming to our class and teaching us about some of the great problems of the world, but most importantly, how we can help. I was really inspired by you, and I really can't wait to get started on my MOGO plan. It was a shocking week for me, but I think that is an important part of educating people about these problems. I would really like to help freetheslaves.net as well as local animal shelters. I have no doubt that last week will stay with me my entire life, and [I] thank you for giving me that experience and the courage to change the world.

• • •

> I want to thank you for teaching us. You gave us so much in such a short time, yet I know I will remember your teaching for a long time. You showed some of the world's problems,

but instead of leaving us in despair, you left us with hope. Much of what you taught us I had no idea of, but the information will definitely influence my choices. Things like the bottled water statistics shocked me. Nevertheless, not drinking bottled water is an easy change to make. Thank you for helping to make the world a better place.

• • •

Thanks so much for coming in to talk to us. It was shocking and inspiring for me. I appreciate what you showed us, especially the movies [*The New Heroes* series]. All of them were really interesting to me. After watching them I realized that it actually was possible to make such a big difference for those who need it most, and that there are people out there who are helping [to] do good right now. After you came in to teach I was opened to a new world of trouble, and new ways to solve and diminish problems. I hung my MOGO plan up on my wall and refer to it whenever I get the time. Thanks again for opening my eyes.

For me, these letters and stories capture the essence of MOGO: willingness to know, commitment to choose wisely and in accordance with our values, and an empowering belief in our capacity to make a difference. And then, when we choose MOGO, what follows is a sense of peace that comes with self-respect, self-acceptance, and responsibilities carried with joy and perseverance.

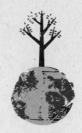

9. The World and You

We all know that the challenges we face in creating a humane, peaceful, and sustainable world are daunting. None of us can individually MOGO our way to a perfect world, and single-handedly solve such problems as global warming, loss of bio-diversity, war, poverty, the energy crisis, and cruelty perpetrated annually upon billions of animals. But together we can solve these and other problems, and the only reason we might not be successful is if too few of us take up this challenge.

By now, I hope I've convinced you that this is not just about doing what's best for the world; it is also about improving your own life in the process. As you embark on the path of MOGO living, your life will become more meaningful, peaceful, enlivened, and purposeful. Others around you will be inspired by your example, and they will join you. Their lives will become more meaningful, too. My hope is that more and more people will form groups that joyfully and tenaciously solve the problems of our time, and more and more communities will strive to do the most good and the least harm. The world will change for the better. We will all be healthier and happier.

This is not a Pollyanna vision. It is absolutely possible.

Philosopher Peter Singer ends his essay "The Good Life" with this:

Anyone can become part of the critical mass that offers us
a chance of improving the world before it is too late ... the
commitment to a more ethical way of living will be the first
step of a gradual but far-reaching evolution in your lifestyle, and in your thinking about your place in the world.
You will take up new causes and find your goals shifting. If
you get involved in your work, money and status will
become less important. From your new perspective, the
world will look different. One thing is certain: you will find
plenty of worthwhile things to do. You will not be bored
or lack fulfillment in your life. Most important of all, you
will know that you have not lived and died for nothing,
because you will have become part of the great tradition
of those who have responded to the amount of pain and
suffering in the universe by trying to make the world a better place.[1]

MOGO living brings about true freedom. When you have the
inner conviction to do the most good and the least harm, you are
free to say no to media, social, and peer pressures. You are free
from a nagging sense that your life does not have value or meaning. You are free to imagine and then create a truly successful (in
the deepest meaning of the word) life. You are free to be at peace
with yourself and all those whom your life touches.

Those striving to lead MOGO lives, who are eagerly involved
in positive change and who consciously make their life their message, are everywhere. They are nurses and architects, students
and teachers, carpenters and physicians, farmers and executives,
plumbers and politicians, factory workers and businesspeople,
engineers and scientists, parents and teenagers, children and senior citizens. They may not yet be the majority, but they can
become the majority if you join them.

In his book *Collapse*, Jared Diamond offers a sobering assess-
ment of the great challenges of our time:

---

1. Peter Singer, *Writings on an Ethical Life* (New York: HarperCollins, 2000), 270–272.

Because we are rapidly advancing along this nonsustainable course, the world's . . . problems will get resolved, in one way or another, within the lifetimes of the children and young adults alive today. The only question is whether they will become resolved in pleasant ways of our own choice or in unpleasant ways not of our choice, such as warfare, genocide, starvation, disease epidemics, and the collapse of societies.[2]

At the end of his exhaustive book, Diamond says that he is cautiously optimistic. So am I. Choosing to solve our most pervasive, dangerous, and escalating problems is a huge challenge, and it is easy to be pessimistic rather than optimistic, but there are good reasons to be confident that we will succeed. First, as Diamond himself points out, we are not facing insoluble problems. We have caused them, and so we can choose to stop causing them and start solving them. Second, as I wrote in the introduction, we humans may have created many problems, but we have also ended a host of atrocities. As Paul Hawken, environmentalist, businessman, and author, says:

The great thing about the dilemma we're in is that we get to re-imagine every single thing we do. . . . There isn't a single thing that doesn't require a complete remake. There are two ways of looking at that. One is: "Oh my gosh, what a big burden." The other way, which I prefer, is: "What a great time to be born! What a great time to be alive!" Because this generation gets to essentially completely change the world.[3]

Human nature may not change much over time. We like our pleasures and our lifestyles; we have difficulty thinking about others too far removed from our inner circle of family, friends, and local community; we are prone to fear difference and be

---

2. Jared Diamond, *Collapse: How Societies Choose to Fail or Succeed* (New York: Viking, 2005), 498.

3. Quoted in Zac Goldsmith's, "You Have Been Warned," *Ecologist* (September, 2007): 32.

territorial; we often think our beliefs are the only ones that are really true and right; we are susceptible to greed and envy. But this is not all that we are. Humans are also altruistic and noble, willing to sacrifice for our ideals, eager to learn and grow, compassionate and generous, and stupendously creative. When we turn our creativity toward the task of a better future for ourselves, for the next generation, and for all life, and when we clarify our values, we can and will make new choices—ones that give us greater peace as we build a peaceful world together. As Ted Nordhaus and Michael Shellenberger write in their book *Break Through: From the Death of Environmentalism to the Politics of Possibility*, "The future is not destined to be dark or bright, fallen or triumphant. Rather, the future is *open*."[4]

And as Frances Moore Lappé writes in her book *Democracy's Edge*, "Our species would never have made it this far if we weren't by nature problem solvers, creatures with a deep need for effectiveness in the wider world. We are most energized when our lives have purpose and meaning."[5] Mix our deep need for effectiveness, and our desire for purpose and meaning, with a commitment to MOGO living, and we have the perfect recipe for the enthusiastic self and societal discipline that are necessary for the tasks before us.

I will leave you with one final quote from children's advocate, Marian Wright Edelman:

"A lot of people are waiting for Martin Luther King Jr. or Mahatma Gandhi to come back, but they are gone. We are it. It is up to us. It is up to you."

---

4. Michael Shellenberger and Ted Nordhaus, *Break Through* (Boston: Houghton Mifflin, 2007), 240.

5. Frances Moore Lappé, *Democracy's Edge* (San Francisco: Jossey-Bass, 2006), 310.

PART III
GETTING STARTED

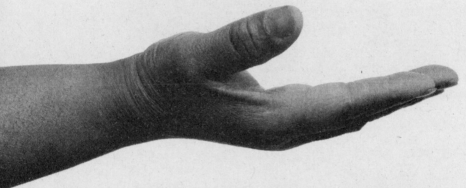

The rest of this book includes a variety of resources, from the **MOGO Questionnaire and Action Plan** that follows, to relevant facts and statistics, to recommended websites, books, periodicals, and videos. This section is integral to this book. I have given you only the briefest information on complicated subjects and issues. To live as MOGO as possible, you'll need to use the 3 Is actively, and this section provides a place to start.

My hope is that I've inspired you to read on, and further your knowledge with passion and commitment. I hope, too, that you will share what you find out with me. As I said in the introduction, I have as much to learn from you as I hope you have to learn from me. I would love to hear your stories, experiences, challenges, and successes in trying to lead a life that does the most good and the least harm.

Zoe Weil
zoe@HumaneEducation.org

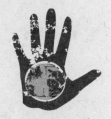

10. MOGO
Questionnaire
and Action Plan

The following questionnaire and action plan gives you the opportunity to reflect upon your choices and your vision for your life, and put into words some concrete goals. As you complete it, try to tap into your deepest wisdom and your most ardent hopes for yourself, your family, your community, and the world we all share.

If you haven't already begun a MOGO journal, now's a good time to start one. Let this questionnaire and action plan launch you on your journey toward MOGO living, serving as a guide to which you can return again and again, and which you can modify and expand with new knowledge, experiences, and understanding.

You'll notice as you complete this questionnaire that most questions are divided into three parts: (a) what you currently do, (b) what you want to learn/do, and (c) what steps you will take. The purpose of this three-part approach is to help you: (a) identify the ways in which you already live according to your values, (b) inquire about what you need to learn to lead a MOGO life, and (c) introspect in order to make tangible plans so that you might live with deeper integrity.

Initially, there may not appear to be much difference between (b) and (c). You'll be asked in (b) to clarify what you think you need to learn, or what you'd like to change. Then you'll be asked in (c) to write down the steps you will take to follow through, and it may seem that you've already done this in (b). But the purpose of the third part of each question is to make very concrete and very manageable plans for yourself. Please make sure to write down only those ideas that are actually possible to carry through, and that truly inspire you.

MOGO Questionnaire and Action Plan

1. The qualities (values) that are most important to me are:

2. **a)** With my family, friends, and neighbors I model the following qualities:

b) I would like to model the following qualities that reflect my values more consciously with my family and friends:

c) In order to achieve this goal, I will take the following steps:

3. **a)** In relation to my health (physical, emotional, intellectual, spiritual) I take care of myself in the following ways:

b) I would like to learn/do the following in order to improve my health (physical, emotional, intellectual, spiritual):

c) I will take the following steps to improve my health (physical, emotional, intellectual, spiritual):

4. a) In relation to people who produce and supply the products and services I use, I currently make the following choices to prevent others from suffering or being exploited:

b) In relation to people who produce and supply the products and services I use, I need to learn about the following in order to make choices that better reflect my values:

c) I will take the following steps to learn, think critically, and make more humane choices in relation to people who produce and supply the products and services I use:

5. a) In relation to animals (wildlife, and those used for food and clothing, in product testing, in forms of entertainment, who are in shelters, and so on), I currently make the following choices to minimize animal suffering and exploitation:

b) In relation to animals (wildlife, and those used for food and clothing, in product testing, in forms of entertainment, who are in shelters, and so on), I need to learn about the following in order to make choices that better reflect my values in relation to animals:

c) I will take the following steps to learn, think critically, and make more humane choices in relation to animals:

6. a) In relation to the environment (air, salt water, fresh water, land, soil, forests, rainforests, natural resources, and so on), I currently make the following choices to live an environmentally friendly, sustainable life:

b) In relation to the environment (air, salt water, fresh water, land, soil, forests, rainforests, natural resources, and so on), I need to learn about the following in order to make choices that better reflect my commitment to protecting and restoring the environment:

c) I will take the following steps to learn, think critically, and make more environmentally friendly, sustainable choices:

7. a) In relation to activism and volunteerism, I already do the following:

b) In relation to activism and volunteerism, I would like to help more in the following ways:

c) I will take the following steps in order to help others through activism and volunteerism:

8. a) In relation to charitable giving and sharing my resources, I contribute in the following ways:

b) In relation to charitable giving and sharing my resources, I would like to contribute more enthusiastically and effectively in these ways:

c) I will take the following steps to contribute more enthusiastically and effectively:

9. a) In relation to democracy, I'm active and engaged in the following ways:

b) In relation to democracy, I need to learn the following in order to be more meaningfully and actively engaged, and participatory:

c) In relation to democracy, I will take the following steps to be more meaningfully and actively engaged in the democratic process:

10. This is the epitaph I would like to have:

11. In order to turn my intentions in this questionnaire into practical changes, I will use the following methods to support and discipline myself (this support can be internal, such as starting a meditation practice; or external, such as taking a class, finding or creating a support group, or a combination of both):

12. Within the next week, I am going to do the following three to five things in order to implement this plan:

13. I am going to put a reminder to myself in my calendar on this date to assess and evaluate my efforts and successes at fulfilling my commitments, and to further evolve my plan:

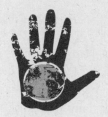

11. Relevant Facts and Statistics

On Food

This chapter contains statistics from John Robbins's book *The Food Revolution: How Your Diet Can Help Save Your Life and the World* related to the effects of animal agriculture on the environment, on world hunger, on human health, and on animals. These statistics aren't meant to take the place of your own research and reading, but if you find them compelling, moving, shocking, or even just interesting, you may want to read Robbins's book.[1] Many of these statistics are based on information from the United States, but since many U.S. companies sell their products across the globe, and since the United States exports not only its products but also its economic systems and political perspectives, these facts and statistics are pertinent indicators for other countries and communities as well.

---

1. While I have not included citations, each statistic is carefully sourced and referenced in John Robbins's book: *The Food Revolution: How Your Diet Can Help Save Your Life and the World* (San Francisco: Conari Press, 2002).

Health

- Percentage of eight-year-old child's daily value for saturated fat in one Burger King Double Whopper with cheese: more than 200
- Percentage of adult daily value for saturated fat in one Double Whopper with Cheese: 130
- Risk of death from heart disease for vegetarians compared to nonvegetarians: half
- Blood cholesterol levels of complete vegetarians (who consume no meat, fish, dairy, or eggs) compared to those of nonvegetarians: 35 percent lower
- Percentage of patients with high blood pressure who are able to completely discontinue use of medications after adopting a low-sodium, low-fat, high-fiber, plant-based diet: 58
- Countries with the highest consumption of dairy products: Finland, Sweden, United States, England
- Countries with the highest rates of osteoporosis: Finland, Sweden, United States, England
- Daily calcium intake for African-Americans: more than 1,000 mg
- Daily calcium intake for black South Africans: 196 mg
- Hip fracture rate for African-Americans compared to that of black South Africans: 9 times greater
- Leading cause of food-borne illness in the United States: Campylobacter bacteria
- Number of people in the United States who become ill with Campylobacter poisoning every day: more than 5,000
- Number of annual Campylobacter-related fatalities in the United States: more than 750
- Primary source of Campylobacter bacteria: contaminated chicken flesh
- Percentage of American chickens sufficiently contaminated with Campylobacter to cause illness: 70
- Percentage of American turkeys sufficiently contaminated with Campylobacter to cause illness: 90

- Number of hens in three commercial flocks screened for Campylobacter by University of Wisconsin researchers: 2,300
- Number of hens *not* infected with Campylobacter: 8
- Number of Americans sickened from eating Salmonella-tainted eggs every year: more than 650,000
- Number of Americans killed from eating Salmonella-tainted eggs every year: 600
- Amount of antibiotics administered to people in the United States annually to treat diseases: 3 million pounds
- Amount of antibiotics administered to livestock in the United States annually for purposes other than treating disease: 24.6 million pounds
- Number of antibiotics allowed in U.S. cow's milk: 80
- Amount of minerals in organic food compared to conventional food:

Calcium	63 percent greater
Chromium	78 percent greater
Iodine	73 percent greater
Iron	59 percent greater
Magnesium	138 percent greater
Potassium	125 percent greater
Selenium	390 percent greater
Zinc	60 percent greater

World Hunger

- Number of people whose food energy needs can be met by the food produced on 2.5 acres of land:

If the land is producing cabbage	23 people
If the land is producing potatoes	22 people
If the land is producing rice	19 people
If the land is producing corn	17 people
If the land is producing wheat	15 people
If the land is producing chicken	2 people
If the land is producing beef	1 person

🌿 Amount of grain needed to adequately feed every person on the entire planet who dies of hunger and hunger-caused diseases annually: 12 million tons

🌿 Percentage by which Americans would have to reduce their beef consumption to save 12 million tons of grain: 10

Environmental Concerns

🌿 Amount of water required to produce 1 pound of California foods, according to soil and water specialists at the University of California Agricultural Extension, working with livestock farm advisors:

1 pound of lettuce	23 gallons/87 liters
1 pound of tomatoes	23 gallons/87 liters
1 pound of potatoes	24 gallons/91 liters
1 pound of wheat	25 gallons/95 liters
1 pound of carrots	33 gallons/125 liters
1 pound of apples	49 gallons/185 liters
1 pound of chicken	815 gallons/3,085 liters
1 pound of pork	1,630 gallons/6,170 liters
1 pound of beef	5,214 gallons/19,737 liters

🌿 Number of calories of fossil fuel expended to produce 1 calorie of protein from soybeans: 2

🌿 Number of calories of fossil fuel expended to produce 1 calorie of protein from corn or wheat: 3

🌿 Number of calories of fossil fuel expended to produce 1 calorie of protein from beef: 54

🌿 Amount of waste (stored in open cesspools) produced by North Carolina's 7 million factory-raised hogs compared to the amount produced by the state's 6.5 million people: 4 to 1

🌿 Relative concentration of pathogens in hog waste compared to human sewage: 10 to 100 times greater

🌿 Total global area planted in genetically engineered crops in 1995: negligible

- Total global area planted in genetically engineered crops in 1999: 99 million acres
- No public records need to be kept of which farms are using genetically engineered seed, and no one needs to label seeds, crops, or food products with information about their genetically engineered origins.

Animal Suffering

- Mass of breast tissue of eight-week-old chicken today compared with 25 years ago: 7 times greater
- Percentage of broiler chickens who are so obese by the age of six weeks that they can no longer walk: 90
- Number of U.S. pigs raised for meat: 90 million per year
- Number of U.S. pigs raised in total confinement factories where they never see the light of day until being trucked to slaughter: 65 million
- Percentage of U.S. pigs who have pneumonia at time of slaughter: 70
- Average number of days newborn calves stay with their mothers: 1
- Cage space provided to each hen used to produce eggs in modern battery-cage facilities: barely more than this book

On Consumerism

The consumerism and cultural facts and statistics in this section are excerpted from *All-Consuming Passion: Waking up from the American Dream* (3rd edition), produced by the New Road Map Foundation and Northwest Environment Watch. To see the entire document with sources and references visit http://www.ecofuture.org/pk/pkar
9506.html. Once again, while these specific statistics are based on information in the United States, the lifestyles, products, and habits of U.S. citizens are being exported across the globe. These sobering

statistics may help people in other countries avoid the pitfalls of U.S. culture while embracing its freedoms and opportunities.

Happiness and Personal Satisfaction

- Percentage rise in per capita income in the United States since 1970: 62
- Percentage *decrease* in quality of life in the United States since 1970, as measured by the Index of Social Health: 51
- Percentage of Americans making over $100,000 a year who agree with the statement, "I cannot afford to buy everything I really need": 26 percent
- Median size of a new house built in the United States:
    1949: 1,100 sq. ft.
    1970: 1,385 sq. ft.
    1996: 1,950 sq. ft.
- Household size in the United States:
    1970: 3.14 persons per household
    1995: 2.65 persons per household
- Between 1990 and 1996, nearly 19 percent of adult Americans made a voluntary lifestyle change that entailed earning less money (not including regularly scheduled retirement). Eighty-five percent are happy about that change. Nearly 50 percent of them made $35,000 or less before their change.

Time, Television, Shopping, and Advertising

- Amount of time the average American will spend watching television commercials: almost 2 years
- Number of high schools in the United States in 1996: 24,000
- Number of shopping centers in the United States in 1996: 42,130
- Number of new toys issued each year by American toymakers: 3,000 to 6,000
- Spending on toy advertising:
    1983: $357 million
    1993: $878 million

Effects on others

- Percentage of world's goods and services consumed by the world's richest 20 percent: 86
- Percentage of world's goods and services consumed by the world's poorest 20 percent: 1.3
- It would take four earths for everybody on the planet to live the lifestyle of North Americans.
- Since 1940, Americans alone have used up as large a share of the earth's mineral resources as all previous humans put together.
- The waste generated each year in the United States would fill a convoy of 10-ton garbage trucks 145,000 miles long (over halfway to the moon).
- Per capita American consumption of sodas in 1989: 47 gallons
- Per capita American consumption of tap water in 1989: 37 gallons
- Total energy consumed in producing a 12-ounce can of diet soda: 2,200 calories
- Total food energy in a 12-ounce can of diet soda: 1 calorie

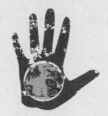

12. Recommended Resources

This list of some of my favorite websites includes portals to helpful information on peaceful and sustainable living; non-profit organizations that attempt to alleviate suffering, raise awareness, prevent destruction, and promote democracy; and businesses that offer humane and sustainable products and services. The inclusion of these particular websites does not imply that they are the only sources of information on these topics; rather, they are meant to get you started without overwhelming you. There is an obvious bias here. If you want corporate and industry perspectives, you can usually go to the website listed on a specific product or find pro-industry sites by simply doing a search on a subject such as "coal," "nuclear energy," "plastics," and so forth.

The Institute for Humane Education (IHE) Website

Websites change all the time. By the time you read this book, some of the websites listed may no longer exist or may have a different URL. For a continually updated list with links, you may wish to go directly to our website at the Institute for Humane Education: HumaneEducation.org. Then go to the resources section, where you'll find up-to-date websites and direct links to them.

Multi-issue Websites for Better Living and a Better World

A Better Future abetterfurture.org
Find out what one person can do to make a difference about a range of issues.

The Breakthrough Institute breakthroughinstitute.org
Here's a small think tank with big ideas for a thriving, safe, healthy world for all.

Care 2 Make a Difference care2.com
As their byline says, "Over 5 million members who care 2 make a difference—Environment, Health, Human Welfare, Animals, Education, Women & More...." Get information and find out what you can do.

Center for a New American Dream newdream.org
From personal choices to activism, you'll find great ideas and information here.

Co-op America coopamerica.org
One of the best sources for learning about virtually all the issues related to humane and sustainable living, this is a website to bookmark!

Earthrights International earthrights.org
Earthrights combines research, education, advocacy, and litigation on behalf of people around the world whose earth rights have been violated by governments and transnational corporations.

Global Exchange globalexchange.org
Find everything from getting involved in human rights work, to travel that helps, to a fair trade store.

Global Issues globalissues.org
Learn much more about many of the issues raised in this book, from human rights, to politics, to trade issues, to health.

I Buy Different   ibuydifferent.org
Find out what happens behind the scenes of everyday purchases, and learn how to shop differently and better.

Responsible Shopper   responsibleshopper.org
This is the easiest way to learn about your products. Look up specific products and companies, and learn about their effects—both positive and negative—on other people, animals, and the environment.

Sustainable Communities Network   sustainable.org
Here's everything you want to know about living sustainably, and creating sustainable communities and events.

Taking It Global   takingitglobal.org
This site empowers young people to learn about issues in the global community and to take positive action.

Wiser Earth   wiserearth.org
This is a community directory and networking forum that maps and connects nongovernmental organizations and individuals addressing the central issues of our day: climate change, poverty, the environment, peace, water, hunger, social justice, conservation, human rights, and more. Content is created and edited by the public.

Human Rights and Social Justice

Anti-Slavery International   antislavery.org
Learn about escalating worldwide slavery and what you can do about it.

Child Labor Coalition   stopchildlabor.org
Find out what's happening to children around the globe, and learn about campaigns to stop child labor.

Ella Baker Center for Human Rights   ellabakercenter.org
A strategy and action center working for justice, opportunity, and peace in urban America, this organization promotes

green-collar jobs and other positive alternatives to violence and incarceration.

Human Rights Watch   hrw.org
Find out about a range of human rights issues and abuses around the world, and what you can do to help.

One World   oneworld.net
Here you'll find extensive information on human rights issues, including campaigns of different organizations.

Environment & Sustainability

David Suzuki Foundation   davidsuzuki.org
This is a solutions-oriented site for environmental sustainability.

Earth Island Institute   earthisland.org
Learn about a variety of environmental issues, subscribe to Earth Island Journal, *get involved, and find out about the Brower Youth Awards.*

Ecological Footprint Quiz   myfootprint.org
Take the ecological footprint quiz, and find out how you can reduce your footprint.

Global Resource Action Center for the
Environment (GRACE)   gracelinks.org
This is a great source of information on critical environmental issues with suggested actions you can take.

Green Dimes   greendimes.com
Stop 90 percent of your junk mail with the help of this site.

Animal Protection

Animal Concerns Community   animalconcerns.org
Go here if you're seeking a clearinghouse for information related to animal rights and welfare.

Animal Legal & Historical
Information Center   animallaw.info
> *Get your U.S. animal law info here, including statutes, full-text cases, articles, topic explorations, and more. The site is searchable by state, subject, and species, and it also includes selected animal laws for twelve other countries.*

Humane Society of the United States   hsus.org
> *Learn the issues related to animal protection, and sign up for action alerts from the largest animal protection organization in the nation.*

People for the Ethical Treatment of Animals   peta.org
> *You'll find no animal left out of this website and will learn more than you can imagine about how you can make a difference for animals.*

World Society for the Protection
of Animals   wspa-international.org
> *This is an international animal welfare organization working all over the world to stop animal abuse.*

Food, Agriculture, and Diet

Center for Food Safety   centerforfoodsafety.org
> *Go here to find out what you need to know about food safety and how you can take action to ensure safe food.*

Food Revolution   foodrevolution.org
> *My favorite book about food has this great accompanying website.*

GoVeg.com   goveg.com
> *Interested in vegetarianism? This is a thorough site on the subject.*

Farmers' Markets   http://www.ams.usda.gov/farmersmarkets
> *Use this resource to find a farmers' market near you.*

Organic Trade Association ota.com
Find out information on organics here.

Pesticide Action Network panna.org
This site details the facts on pesticides—what you should know and what you can do.

True Food Shoppers Guide http://www.truefoodnow.org/shoppersguide
Go here to learn about which products and brands are genetically engineered.

Media

Commercial Alert commercialalert.org
Learn how to get involved with keeping commercial culture in its place.

Campaign for a Commercial-Free
Childhood commercialexploitation.com
As the name implies, find out how to stop harmful marketing to children.

Media Foundation adbusters.org
Find innovative ideas for challenging the commercialized world, from cutting-edge commentary to creative spoof ads.

Humane Education

Americans Who Tell the Truth americanswhotellthetruth.org
Artist Robert Shetterly has been painting portraits of Americans who tell the truth, from historical heroes to current activists. This series, captured in his book by the same title, also comes with curricula for teachers.

The Big Picture Company bigpicture.org
The BPC strives to "catalyze vital changes in American education by generating and sustaining innovative, personalized

schools that work in tandem with the real world of their greater community." Find out how they're doing it.

Cloud Institute for Sustainability
Education   sustainabilityed.org
The Cloud Institute works with K–12 schools to bring concepts of sustainability to students and create a sustainable world.

Educators for Social Responsibility   esrnational.org
This organization offers lessons and activities about social justice issues, has a magazine, and offers other support for educators and schools.

Green Teacher   greenteacher.com
Learn about the magazine and online articles, and related activities for teachers.

The Hero Workshop   thejanuscenter.com/heroworkshop/
This workshop and curriculum enables young people to learn about heroic acts, heroic people, and most importantly to cultivate ordinary heroism.

Humane Education Advocates Reaching
Teachers (HEART)   teachhumane.org
HEART's goal is to infuse all educational settings with humane education. Find resources for teachers at their site.

Institute for Humane Education   HumaneEducation.org
This is the organization I cofounded. Download humane education lesson plans and activities; participate in an online course; and/or learn about our Master of Education degree program, certificate program, and workshops.

Rethinking Schools   rethinkingschools.org
Go to this online version of the magazine by the same name, with publications, links, and other resources for promoting social justice issues among youth.

Roots and Shoots   rootsandshoots.org
   Explore Jane Goodall's humane education program, which
   reaches thousands of children, and find out how you can
   bring Roots and Shoots to your local schools.

Teaching Tolerance   teachingtolerance.org
   This organization provides educational materials for promot-
   ing "respect for differences and appreciation for diversity."

Youth for Environmental Sanity (YES!)   yesworld.org
   YES! programs help youth become engaged and involved in
   healthy, positive change-making for the good of all.

Political Reform and Democracy

Accurate Democracy   accuratedemocracy.com
   This is the site for learning about democracy.

Center for Responsive Politics   opensecrets.org
   Find out where the money comes from and how it goes back
   into politics.

Center for Voting and Democracy   fairvote.org
   Learn about the solution of Instant Runoff Voting.

Common Cause   commoncause.org
   Find out how to promote democracy and clean up Congress.

Congress   congress.org
   If you live in the United States, just visit this site and plug in
   your zip code to contact your legislators, and read their posi-
   tions and other commentaries.

New America Foundation   newamerica.net
   Read about suggested policies and solutions to common politi-
   cal issues and concerns.

Service Organizations

Lions Club International   lionsclub.org
Lions is currently the largest service club doing both local and global work to make a difference. There are Lions clubs in most communities.

Rotary International   rotaryinternational.org
An international service club whose motto is "service above self," Rotary is the world's first service club, and works both locally and globally. There are Rotary Clubs in most communities.

Business for a Better World

BuildingGreen, Inc.   buildinggreen.com
Here's where you go when you need to know about building sustainably and safely.

Drop Soul   dropsoul.com
This is a helpful site for environmental, fair trade, and cruelty-free products.

Freecycle   freecycle.org
The site for giving away and getting free stuff.

The Green Guide   thegreenguide.com
Find lots of information on green living, including Community-Supported Agriculture (CSA farms), near you.

Green Home Environmental Store   greenhome.com
Find eco-friendly products in many categories: clothes, appliances, furniture, and more.

Healthy Building Network   healthybuilding.net
Find out what you need to know to build sustainably and safely.

Idealist.org   idealist.org
Go here for jobs, opportunities, and events geared toward people who want to make a difference.

Real Goods   realgoods.com
Find everything here, from organic cotton to solar, off-the-grid living.

Sustainable Business E-newsletter   sustainablebusiness.com
This is an e-newsletter full of information on sustainable business, green jobs, legislation, and breaking news.

Vegan Essentials   veganessentials.com
A cruelty-free online store.

Working Assets   workingassets.com
Provides credit cards and long distance phone service, and donates a portion of profits to nonprofits working for a better world.

Zipcar   zipcar.com
Depending upon what city you live in, this site offers an affordable and practical alternative to urban car ownership, letting you have access to a car when you need it.

Community-Building, Volunteering, and Sharing

Conversation Café   conversationcafe.org
Find a conversation café near you, meet interesting people concerned with some of the same issues raised in this book, and start talking!

Meet Up   meetup.com
Find people near you with whom you can learn something, do something, share something, or change something.

Neighborrow   neighborrow.com
Meet, borrow, share, and trade with neighbors.

Time Banks   timebanks.org
The mission of Time Banks is to strengthen communities through reciprocity.

Volunteer Match   volunteermatch.org
Find out about volunteer opportunities in your neighborhood.

Travel/Volunteer Opportunities

Amizade   amizade.org
Volunteer in building construction, tutoring, and food distribution overseas to help others in need.

Cross-Cultural Solutions   crossculturalsolutions.org
At this site, you'll find a variety of volunteer opportunities lasting two to twelve weeks in a range of countries.

Earthwatch Institute   earthwatch.org
Volunteer on ecological and wildlife projects around the world.

Global Volunteers   globalvolunteers.org
This is another program that provides the opportunity to volunteer overseas and help others.

Investing and Finances

Co-op America Greenpages   http://www.coopamerica.org/
                                pubs/greenpages
For information on ethical financing, scroll to the many topics under "financial."

Credit Unions   creditunion.coop
Information on member-owned credit unions near you.

Kiva   kiva.org
Although you won't make money on your investment with Kiva, you'll be helping people caught in poverty to break the cycle through small loans.

Social Investment Forum   socialinvest.org
Here's an association dedicated to advancing the concept, practice, and growth of socially and environmentally responsible investing (SRI).

Conferences and Festivals

Bioneers   bioneers.org
> *This three-day annual conference in San Rafael, California, beamed by satellite all over the world, brings together change-makers and problem-solvers to discuss a range of issues— environment, sustainability, humane living, peace and justice, and human rights.*

Green Festivals   greenfestivals.org
> *Green Fests are offered at several cities in the United States, bringing together speakers, booths, green businesses and products, and networking opportunities for those interested in the interrelated issues of sustainability, environmentalism, human rights, animal protection, and peace. Green Fests are sponsored by Global Exchange and Co-op America.*

Recommended Books

Below are some of my top picks of books to read to further your education, but this list is by no means complete. To find a full listing of frequently updated recommended books, visit Humane Education.org.

Books Covering a Variety of Issues Related to Humane and Sustainable Living and Creating a Better World

Above All, Be Kind: Raising a Humane Child in Challenging Times, by Zoe Weil, New Society Publishers, 2003.
> *This is my book for parents who want to raise humane children.*

Break Through: From the Death of Environmentalism to the Politics of Possibility, by Ted Nordhaus and Michael Shellenberger, Houghton Mifflin, 2007.
> *Explore one of the most important, visionary books for people who want to create meaningful, visionary change on behalf of all and reject the politics of fear.*

Capitalism 3.0: A Guide to Reclaiming the Commons, by Peter Barnes, Berrett-Koehler, 2006.
Here's a compelling case for a modified capitalism in which we protect our collective commons and further prosperity.

Cradle to Cradle: Remaking the Way We Make Things, by William McDonough and Michael Braungart, North Point Press, 2002.
Read this book! You'll be inspired and delighted about the future we can create.

Creating a World that Works for All, by Sharif Abdullah, Berrett-Koehler, 1999.
This is a powerful book packed with vision and ideas for creating a better world.

The Culture of Make Believe, by Derrick Jensen, Context Books, 2002.
Discover one of the most exhaustive books about the interconnected problems not only of our time but throughout history. Depressing but illuminating, this book can lay the groundwork for visionary books such as, Break Through *and* Cradle to Cradle.

Democracy's Edge: Choosing to Save our Country by Bringing Democracy to Life, by Frances Moore Lappé, Jossey-Bass, 2006.
I've already referred to this book repeatedly. It's a must-read for those wanting to engage in democracy.

Field Notes on the Compassionate Life, by Marc Ian Barasch, Rodale, 2005.
Here's a volume of one story after another that will amaze and inspire you.

Stuff: The Secret Lives of Everyday Things, by Alan Thein Durning and John C. Ryan, Northwest Environment Watch, 1997.
You'll never look at stuff the same way again after you read this gem of a little book that's packed with information.

The Third Side, by William Ury, Penguin Books, 1999.
This book provides the framework for solving conflicts and seeking out more than either/or answers to problems.

Voluntary Simplicity, by Duane Elgin, William Morrow, 1993.
 This is the book that launched the movement.

Writings on an Ethical Life, by Peter Singer, HarperCollins, 2000.
 Read this powerful call to ethical living covering a variety of moral issues.

Human Rights

Confessions of an Economic Hit Man, by John Perkins, Berrett-Koehler, 2004.
 Brace yourself for this best-selling exposé of corrupt and destructive systems that's as riveting as any mystery.

Crossing the Boulevard: Strangers, Neighbors, Aliens in a New America, by Judith Sloan and Warren Lehrer, Norton, 2003.
 Funny, sad, powerful, moving—this book is a celebration of immigrant stories.

Ending Slavery, by Kevin Bales, University of California Press, 2007.
 This book pulls back the curtain on escalating worldwide slavery, and provides many examples and ideas for eradicating it.

Faces of Racism, by Joseph Szwarc, Amnesty International, 2001.
 Explore this short, powerful introduction to the many forms of bigotry in our world.

Free the Children, by Craig Kielburger, HarperPerennial, 1998.
 This is one of the most inspiring examples of what a young person can accomplish, complete with what you need to know about child slavery and child labor.

The Lucifer Effect, by Philip Zimbardo, Random House, 2007.
 Witness an in-depth discussion of the infamous Stanford Prison Experiment that provides a paradigm for thinking about change that takes into consideration the person, the situation, and the system.

Material World: A Global Family Portrait, by Peter Menzel, Sierra Club Books, 1994.
 A pictorial account of what average families from different countries own, this is the most important coffee table book ever.

Environmental Issues

Choose to Reuse, by Nikki and David Goldbeck, Ceres Press, 1995.
Discover a goldmine of suggestions.

Collapse: How Societies Choose to Fail or Succeed, by Jared Diamond, Viking, 2005.
Thorough, fascinating, and scholarly yet readable, this book is a combination of history, sociology, anthropology, science, and a compelling call to action.

Gone Tomorrow: The Hidden Life of Garbage, by Heather Rogers, The New Press, 2005.
Ever wonder where our garbage goes? Find out in this well-researched book.

The Last Hours of Ancient Sunlight, by Thom Hartmann, Mythical Books, 1998.
This is one of those books that puts together many pieces of the puzzle of today's challenges.

Our Ecological Footprint, by Mathis Wackernagel and William Rees, New Society Publishers, 1996.
Presented here is a system for analyzing the effects of one's choices on the environment.

Silent Spring, by Rachel Carson, Houghton Mifflin, 1962.
The classic that launched the environmental movement, this is a must read.

Animal Issues

Animal Liberation, by Peter Singer, Avon, 1975.
This is the book that launched the animal rights movement and is the most important on the subject ever written—another must read.

Building an Ark: 101 Solutions to Animal Suffering, by Ethan Smith with Guy Dauncey, New Society Publishers, 2007.
Covering the range of ways in which we use animals and cause them to suffer, this book offers practical ways to stop animal suffering.

Claude and Medea: The Hellburn Dogs, by Zoe Weil, Lantern Books, 2007.
This is the first novel in a children's series (for ages eight to twelve) about seventh-grade clandestine activists in New York City who are inspired by an eccentric substitute teacher to rescue stolen dogs from a laboratory.

The Dreaded Comparison, by Marjorie Spiegel, Mirror Books, 1997.
This is a thought-provoking comparison between human and animal slavery.

The Emotional Lives of Animals, by Marc Bekoff, PhD, New World Library, 2007.
As the title implies, this book, written by an ethologist, examines animal emotions and recounts beautiful, compelling accounts of animals' ability to feel.

Slaughterhouse, by Gail Eisnetz, Prometheus Books, 1997.
Don't let the title scare you away. Everyone should take the time to read this book.

So, You Love Animals: An Action-Packed, Fun-Filled Book to Help Kids Help Animals, by Zoe Weil, Animalearn, 1994.
I wrote this book for children ages eight to eleven who want to help animals.

Media and Consumer Issues

Affluenza: The All-Consuming Epidemic, by John De Graaf, David Wann, and Thomas H. Naylor, Berrett-Koehler, 2001.
Enjoy this terrific book that looks at modern-day consumerism.

Consuming Kids: The Hostile Takeover of Childhood, by Susan Linn, The New Press, 2004.
This is a very important book about the effects of consumerism on children.

Marketing Madness, by Michael Jacobson and Laurie Ann Mazur, Westview Press, 1995.
Photos, examples, stories—it is a fantastic introduction to the effects of marketing.

No Logo, by Naomi Klein, Picador, 1999.
Branding takes on new meaning in this fascinating book.

The Plug-In Drug, by Marie Winn, Penguin Books, 1985.
What you didn't want to know about the effects of television— this book was written twenty years ago but is still relevant.

Toxic Sludge Is Good for You, by John Stauber and Sheldon Rampton, Common Courage Press, 1995.
Witty and shocking, here's a must-read primer on public relations.

When Corporations Rule the World, by David Korten, Kumarian Press, 1995.
This book presents an instructive lens through which to look at corporations and is written by a former World Bank employee.

Humane Education

The Big Picture: Education is Everyone's Business, by Dennis Littky, ASCD, 2002.
If you're interested in a new paradigm for schools, you should read this book.

Dumbing Us Down, by John Taylor Gatto, New Society Publishers, 1992.
A short treatise, powerfully articulated, by a former teacher of the year in New York City, this book is about what's wrong with our schools.

Earth Education: A New Beginning, by Steve Van Matre, Institute for Earth Education, 1990.
Here's my pick for the best environmental education curriculum.

Earth in Mind, by David Orr, Island Press, 1994.
This is a must-read for every educator.

Educating for Character: How Our Schools Can Teach Respect and Responsibility, by Thomas Likona, Bantam, 1991.
Here's a classic on character education.

Educating for Human Greatness, by Lynn Stoddard, Holistic Education Press, 2003.
This short, inspiring book seeks to fulfill its title.

The Power and Promise of Humane Education, by Zoe Weil, New Society Publishers, 2004.
This is my book for teachers and activists wanting to learn how to offer humane education (complete with activities and lessons).

Rethinking Globalization: Teaching for Justice in an Unjust World, by Bill Bigelow and Bob Peterson, Rethinking Schools Press, 2002.
Chock full of lesson plans and activities, this book is for teachers who want to teach about issues of economic globalization and its effects on others.

Sharing Nature with Children, by Joseph Cornell, Dawn Publications, 1979.
Here's a book brimming with wonderful activities for bringing nature to children and children to nature.

Food and Diet

Diet for a Dead Planet: How the Food Industry is Killing Us, by Christopher D. Cook, The New Press, 2004.
This is everything you should know about the food industry and its effects.

Eat Here: Reclaiming Homegrown Pleasures in a Global Super-market, by Brian Halweil, W. W. Norton, 2004.
This book offers myriad reasons why we should strive to eat local foods.

The Food Revolution, by John Robbins, Conari Press, 2002.
I think this is the most important book on food ever written—a must read.

Harvest for Hope: A Guide to Mindful Eating, by Jane Goodall, Warner Books, 2005.
Beautifully written with moving stories, Jane Goodall's book gives us the recipe for a sustainable, healthy, and humane way of eating.

The Way We Eat: Why Our Food Choices Matter, by Peter Singer and Jim Mason, Rodale, 2006.
This readable and fascinating book answers the question "What are the true costs of our daily food choices?"

Cookbooks

Complete Vegetarian Kitchen, by Lorna Sass, Hearst Books, 1992.
This is my favorite cookbook.

Ecological Cooking, by Joanne Stepaniak and Kathy Hecker, Book Publishing Co., 1991.
This book serves up loads of easy-to-follow recipes.

How It All Vegan, by Tanya Barnard and Sarah Kramer, Arsenal Pulp Press, 2000.
Fun, simple recipes from two rockin' gals.

La Dolce Vegan, by Sarah Kramer, Arsenal Pulp Press, 2005.
An awesome follow-up cookbook to How it All Vegan.

Sweet and Natural, by Meredith McCarthy, St. Martins Press, 1999.
I have three words to say about this book: healthy, delicious desserts!

The Uncheese Cookbook, by Joanne Stepaniak, Book Publishing Co.,1994.
Although this cookbook was recommended to me, I was not especially interested in a cookbook with just cheese alternatives. I got it anyway, and I'm so glad. It's my second-most-used cookbook.

Recommended Periodicals

The Atlantic Monthly—multi-issue, well-researched, thoughtful, and thought-provoking articles

E Magazine—a great environmental magazine that makes connections between the environment, people, and animals

Earth Island Journal—the publication of the Earth Island Institute, this journal is chock full of actions, campaigns, and ways to get involved.

Ecologist—named Environmental Magazine of the Year; a UK publication

Greater Good Magazine—a publication of the Greater Good Science Center at the University of California at Berkeley that explores how to contribute to the greater good of all

Mother Jones—investigative journalism that has been exposing corruption, and oppressive and destructive systems for years

Orion—a gorgeous magazine filled with essays and articles that are moving, educational, holistic, and inspiring

The Sun—the essays, interviews, fiction, and poetry in this magazine are among the most powerful, moving, and instructive.

Yes! A Journal of Positive Futures—as the name implies, a fantastic journal that's helping create a better world; a very worthwhile subscription

*Veg*News*—a beautiful publication for those interested in a vegetarian diet and animal-friendly lifestyle

World Watch—the publication of the Worldwatch Institute, and the best magazine for environmental and sustainability information

Recommended Films

Some of these films are available in multiple formats. For a frequently updated list of recommended movies, please visit the resources section at HumaneEducation.org.

For selections of films on human rights, social justice, and environmental issues, visit:

Bullfrog Films	bullfrogfilms.com
The Film Connection	thefilmconnection.org
News Reel	newsreel.org
Video Project	videoproject.com
YouTube	youtube.com

For selections of films on media issues:

Media Education Foundation	mediaed.org

For selections of films on animal issues:

Farm Sanctuary	farmsanctuary.org
People for the Ethical Treatment of Animals	peta-online.org
Tribe of Heart	tribeofheart.org

Specific recommendations

(To find these films, Google the titles or ask your local library to purchase them.)

The 11th Hour—the huge challenges we face along with suggestions for solving them

Affluenza—an instructive, sobering, yet funny look at materialism in America

An Inconvenient Truth—Al Gore's slide show turned movie about global warming

Blue Vinyl—a quirky, funny, fascinating "true cost" documentary of PVC vinyl

Breaking Barriers—a shocking undercover look inside a primate research facility

Cheap Tricks—behind the scenes of animal entertainment, narrated by Alec Baldwin

Classroom Cut-Ups—an undercover investigation of the two largest biological supply companies that supply animals used in dissection

The Corporation—a brilliant, feature-length look at corporations

Diet for A New America—based on the book by John Robbins, a look at how our food choices affect our health, animals, and the environment

For the Bible Tells Me So—a documentary on homophobia and religious perspectives on homosexuality

The Future of Food—a powerful look at GMOs, focusing on Monsanto's lawsuit against Canadian farmer, Percy Schmeiser, whose crops were contaminated by Monsanto's patented seed

Inside Biosearch—another undercover investigation, this time of an animal testing laboratory in Philadelphia

Killing Us Softly 3—funny, shocking, and sobering, this narrated slide show exposes the media's objectification of women

Making a Killing: Philip Morris, Kraft and the Global Tobacco Addiction—the title speaks for itself

McLibel: The People Who Wouldn't Say Sorry—a documentary about the record-breaking trial of two activists who spoke out against McDonald's

Meet Your Meat—what really happens behind the scenes in meat production

The New Heroes—an inspiring PBS series about fourteen individuals who are making a difference

Peaceable Kingdom—a beautifully produced and powerful look at animal agriculture

Ryan's Well—a young boy learns about the lack of water in an African village, raises funds to build a well, and launches a movement

Sea of Slaughter—based on Farley Mowat's book about the destruction of North Atlantic marine life in last two centuries

Stolen Childhoods—child labor and slavery around the globe

Super Size Me—a feature-length, shocking, funny, and powerful look at what a McDonald's diet did to one man's health

This Is What Democracy Looks Like—a documentary of the Seattle WTO protests

Tough Guise—the damage media is doing to boys and men

Toxic Sludge Is Good for You—public relations and its insidious effects

The True Cost of Food—a brilliant, ten-minute, animated look at the true cost of food

Unnecessary Fuss—stolen footage of head injury experiments on baboons filmed by the researchers themselves; profoundly shocking

Wal-Mart: The High Cost of Low Price—a riveting, feature-length documentary of the effects of Wal-Mart on its own employees, foreign producers of its products, and the environment

The Witness—a powerful documentary of one man's change; moving and meaningful

Acknowledgments

I always find the acknowledgments to be the most personally compelling yet challenging task of any book I write. There are too many people to thank by name, yet I must name names. But before I do, I wish to acknowledge all the writers, thinkers, activists, changemakers, and teachers who have influenced, inspired, and taught me. If this book is of any value, it's because of all those from whom I've learned so much.

Now to the names.

Mary Ann Naples of the Creative Culture is my fantastic agent and my friend. I feel so lucky to have been referred to her long ago by another friend, publishing advisor, and publisher, Martin Rowe. Mary Ann, you do so much more than represent me; you guide my writing with wisdom, clarity, and honesty, and I'm enormously grateful to you.

Everyone at Beyond Words, from publisher Cynthia Black to Marie Hix, Julie Knowles, Lindsay Brown, Courtney Dunham, and Richard Cohn, has been so great to work with. I was utterly delighted to have a conference call with the entire staff early on in this process, and to discover that this is a publishing company with such dedicated personnel—all eager and enthusiastic about the books they are bringing to the world. It's an honor to be one of your authors.

Many people read early drafts of this book, and their honest feedback has helped make the book so much better. Of course, as all authors must tell you, the mistakes lie with me; the ways in which this book is worthy and much improved lie with them. So a huge thank you to: Edwin Barkdoll, Kyle Bissell, Mary Pat Champeau, Dani Dennenberg, Melissa Feldman, Bruce Friedrich,

Roberto Giannicola, Caryn Ginsberg, Steve Gross, Kathy Kandzi-olka, Cari MacDonald, Betsy Pal, Marsha Rakestraw, Matt Wild-man, and Khalif Williams.

I work with the best staff and board I could ever hope for. They are my dear friends and MOGO role models, and I admire each of them enormously. We are led by our outstanding executive director, Khalif Williams. You now know him (from **Key 1—Live Your Epitaph**) as a paragon of MOGOhood; I know him as a both a great leader and close friend. Our Master of Education program is directed by our wise, witty, generous Mary Pat Champeau, without whom I would be both immeasurably less good and less happy. Amy Morley, our operations and events manager, could not possibly be more helpful, dedicated, or kind even if she were a clone of Mother Teresa. Our brilliant and beloved "mama cat," Marsha Rakestraw, makes everything possible through our website and newsletter and personally helps me enormously. Melissa Feldman, my wonderful colleague and close friend for twenty years, and now on our faculty (and whom you also now know from **Key 1—Live Your Epitaph**), continues to teach and inspire me. Our part-time workshop facilitators, Kim Korona and Freeman Wicklund, are so extraordinary I hope you will attend one of their workshops and see for yourself. As you know from my profile of her in **Key 1—Live Your Epitaph**, Kim has been my role model for kindness since I met her. Freeman is just about everyone's role model for good-natured humor no matter what. Several employees have recently left the Institute for Humane Education (IHE): Dani Dennenberg, Carrol Lange, Cari MacDonald, and Kathy Kandziolka. They may have left IHE, but these exceptional women will always be my deeply admired colleagues and friends. Finally, a special thanks to our wonderful volunteer board members: Sheb Bishop, Callie Curtis, Caryn Ginsberg, Kristin Hegazy, and Chick Rauch. IHE continues to grow and achieve its mission largely because of you.

Special thanks to MJ Ryan for consulting with me on the title; to John Robbins for his continuing support and willingness—always—to read my work; and to Steve Piersanti for his interest, encouragement, support, and thoughtful feedback. I met Phil Zimbardo in time to bring his brilliant insights and life's work to this book, and I'm so grateful for his friendship and sharing of ideas during this past year.

Thank you to Rabbi Michael Skobac and Rabbi Mat Hoffman who long ago planted the seeds that led to the MOGO principle.

A very special thanks to Ian Chittenden. While I have been home, writing and working at IHE, my son has been in your classroom, learning from a master humane educator who is a role model for me as both a teacher and as a human being. Teachers (and people) just don't come better than you, Ian.

Steve Komie and Kumara Siddhartha: what you've both done to advance humane education is incalculable. I cannot thank you enough. You will continue to see the fruits.

So much gratitude to my Aikido sensei, David Hill. David, I've learned so much more than Aikido from you. You embody the essence of Aikido in all aspects of your life, and while it would be nice to one day earn my black belt, I care much more about one day being as good, positive, and joyful as you.

I am lucky to have an incredible community of friends, and am so grateful to all of you who have patiently indulged my many questions, listened to my ideas, hiked up Blue Hill and the mountains in Acadia National Park with me, shared meals, and offered your thoughts, feedback, and support. I will not risk leaving out any names by naming you—you know who you are.

Finally, my family. My mother, Peggy Weil, and brother, Stanley Weil III, may not have predicted my particular career path or chosen lifestyle, but they have shown nothing but support for and belief in me and my work, and I'm grateful to both of them. My father, Stanley Weil Jr., who died when I was twenty-three, still continues to guide me. His pure, unconditional, and undemanding love is a thing I've yet to live up to, but I will always try. My memories of my wonderful dad inspire me to be kinder, more loving, more MOGO.

My husband, Edwin Barkdoll, continues to teach me to be a better, clearer thinker. He's both rigorous and relaxed, a delightful mix. I love our conversations, especially our long Wednesday ones, where I get to explore the ideas that wind up in my books. Thank you, Edwin, for your love, support, constancy, and humor.

Acknowledgments

My son, Forest Barkdoll-Weil, is awesome. Forest, I so admire your beautiful combination of generosity and compassion with forthrightness and strength of will. These are MOGO qualities I seek to emulate.

It may not be customary to thank one's animals (especially because omitting them would hardly cause hurt feelings), but I feel compelled to acknowledge our three dogs, Griffin, Sophie, and Ruby, and one cat, Sir Simon. I work from my desk in my bedroom, and these animals are a frequent reminder of the qualities I consider MOGO. The dogs are all deeply loyal, eminently patient, fun-loving, and good-spirited, and they know how to play fair and make amends when they cause harm by mistake. They are irrepressibly enthusiastic about life, and they bear their pains without complaint. Sir Simon, well, he's the king of our household: dignified, unflappable, and calm. I'm grateful to these animals, not only for reminders of MOGO qualities but because I periodically paused during the writing of this book to pet them or take a walk with them, and it is during those times I often pulled my thoughts together and felt the touch of grace that gave me a new idea or understanding that I could share with you.

Which leads me to you. Thanks for all you do now and for all you will continue to do, throughout your life, to make this world better.

About the Institute for Humane Education

The Institute for Humane Education (IHE) works to create a humane world through education. Committed to making living ethically, sustainably, and peaceably on this planet the very purpose of education, IHE trains people to be humane educators, offers workshops and programs on humane education and MOGO living, and advances comprehensive humane education worldwide. Humane education not only inspires individuals to make personal choices that do the most good and the least harm, but it also teaches people how to become critical thinkers and problem solvers who have the knowledge and commitment to pursue creative answers to entrenched global challenges.

In 1997, IHE established the first Humane Education Certificate Program (HECP) in the United States, and in 2000, affiliated with Cambridge College to offer a distance-learning Master of Education degree in humane education (also a first in the United States). IHE offers its acclaimed weekend workshops in the United States and Canada, and each year trains hundreds of people to be humane educators, who in turn reach thousands of students. IHE also offers MOGO workshops and classes designed to educate and empower people to put their values into action in all aspects of their lives and work, and to put the concepts in this book into practice.

To learn more, please visit HumaneEducation.org or email info@HumaneEducation.org.

About the Author

Zoe Weil is the cofounder and president of the Institute for Humane Education (IHE). A humane educator since 1985, Zoe now trains others through the IHE/Cambridge College Master of Education in humane education, IHE's Humane Education Certificate Program, and IHE's workshops and classes. She speaks widely on humane education and MOGO living, and is recognized as a pioneer in comprehensive humane education. She is the author of *Above All, Be Kind: Raising a Humane Child in Challenging Times*; *The Power and Promise of Humane Education*; *So, You Love Animals: An Action-Packed, Fun-Filled Book to Help Kids Help Animals*; and *Claude and Medea: The Hellburn Dogs*, the first in a children's series about twelve-year-old activists.

Zoe received a Master of Theological Studies degree from Harvard Divinity School and a Master of Arts in English Literature from the University of Pennsylvania, and is certified in Psychosynthesis, a form of counseling that relies on individuals' innate wisdom to promote health and well-being.

Zoe lives with her family in coastal Maine. You can contact her at zoe@HumaneEducation.org and read her blog at www.zoe weil.com.

Connect!

Find others who want to learn more and work with you. If you have found this book in a library, add your name and email address below, and contact others who have done the same. If you own this book, write down your name and contact info, and then lend it to others. Or consider donating it to the library when you're done with it.

Name   Email

_____

_____

_____

_____

_____

_____

_____

_____

_____

_____